Neonatal Medications and Procedures

(NEOMAP)

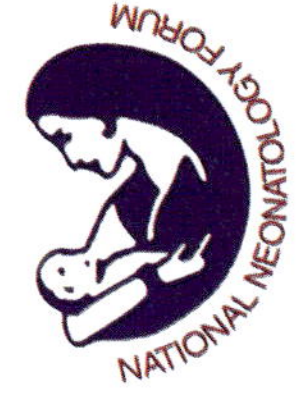

National Neonatology Forum of India

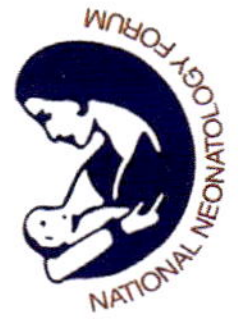

Neonatal Medications and Procedures (NEOMAP)

Editors

Amit Upadhyay
MD (Pediatrics) DM (Neonatology)
Director and Head
Department of Pediatrics and
Neonatology
Nutema Hospital
Meerut, Uttar Pradesh, India
Treasurer (2022–2024)
National Neonatology Forum
National Coordinator, NEOMAP

Sushma Nangia
MD (Pediatrics) DM (Neonatology-AIIMS)
Director–Professor and Head
Department of Neonatology
Lady Hardinge Medical College
and Associated Kalawati Saran
Children Hospital
New Delhi, India

Pratima Anand
MD (Pediatrics) DM (Neonatology)
Consultant Neonatologist
Department of Neonatology
Lady Hardinge Medical College
and Associated Hospitals
New Delhi, India
National Co-ordinator, NEOMAP

Surender Singh Bisht
MD (Pediatrics) DNB (Pediatrics)
Head and Senior Specialist
Department of Pediatrics
Swami Dayanand Hospital
New Delhi, India

Forewords
Siddharth Ramji
Praveen Kumar
Dinesh Tomar

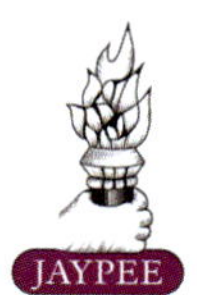

JAYPEE BROTHERS MEDICAL PUBLISHERS

The Health Sciences Publisher

New Delhi | London

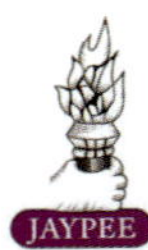 **Jaypee Brothers Medical Publishers (P) Ltd**

Headquarters

Jaypee Brothers Medical Publishers (P) Ltd
EMCA House, 23/23-B
Ansari Road, Daryaganj
New Delhi 110 002, India
Landline: +91-11-23272143, +91-11-23272703
+91-11-23282021, +91-11-23245672
Email: jaypee@jaypeebrothers.com

Corporate Office

Jaypee Brothers Medical Publishers (P) Ltd
4838/24, Ansari Road, Daryaganj
New Delhi 110 002, India
Phone: +91-11-43574357
Fax: +91-11-43574314
Email: jaypee@jaypeebrothers.com

Overseas Office

JP Medical Ltd
83 Victoria Street, London
SW1H 0HW (UK)
Phone: +44 20 3170 8910
Fax: +44 (0)20 3008 6180
Email: info@jpmedpub.com

Website: www.jaypeebrothers.com
Website: www.jaypeedigital.com

Neonatal Medications and Procedures (NEOMAP)

First Edition: **2025**

ISBN: 978-93-5696-461-7

Printed in India at Sterling Graphics Pvt. Ltd.

Contributors

Aakash Pandita
MD (Pediatrics) DrNB (Neonatology)
Medanta Hospital
Lucknow, Uttar Pradesh, India

Amanpreet Sethi
MD (Pediatrics) DM (Neonatology)
Government Medical College
Faridkot, Punjab, India

Amit Upadhyay
MD (Pediatrics) DM (Neonatology)
Nutema Hospital
Meerut, Uttar Pradesh, India
Treasurer (2022–2024)
National Neonatology Forum
National Coordinator, NEOMAP

Anita Singh MD (Pediatrics)
DrNB (Neonatology)
Sanjay Gandhi Postgraduate Institute
of Medical Sciences
Lucknow, Uttar Pradesh, India

Ankit Verma MD (Pediatrics)
All India Institute of Medical Sciences
New Delhi, India

Anu Sachdeva
MD (Pediatrics) DM (Neonatology)
All India Institute of Medical Sciences
New Delhi, India

Aparna C
MD (Pediatrics) DM (Neonatology)
KIMS Cuddles
Hyderabad, Telangana, India

Arjit Mohapatra
MD (Pediatrics) DM (Neonatology)
Jagannath Hospital
Bhubaneswar, Odisha, India

Ashish Jain
MD (Pediatrics) DM (Neonatology)
Maulana Azad Medical College
New Delhi, India

Ashish Mehta MD (Pediatrics)
Arpan Hospital
Ahmedabad, Gujarat, India

Ashok Kumar MD (Pediatrics)
Banaras Hindu University
Varanasi, Uttar Pradesh, India

Ashok Mittal MD (Pediatrics)
Narayan Memorial Hospital
Kolkata, West Bengal, India

Ashwani Singal
MD (Pediatrics) DM (Neonatology)
Sapling Hospital
Ludhiana, Punjab, India

Bijan Saha
MD (Pediatrics) DM (Neonatology)
Institute of Postgraduate Medical
Education and Research and Seth
Sukhlal Karnani Memorial Hospital
Kolkata, West Bengal, India

Chandra Kumar
MD (Pediatrics) DM (Neonatology)
Kanchi Kamakoti CHILDS Trust Hospital
Chennai, Tamil Nadu, India

Deepak Chawla
MD (Pediatrics) DM (Neonatology)
Government Medical College
Chandigarh, India

Dinesh Chirla
MD (Pediatrics) DM (Neonatology)
FRCPCH (UK) Neonatal Fellow (Australia)
Specialist in Neonatology (CCST, UK)
Rainbow Children's Hospital
Hyderabad, Telangana, India

Jagjit Dalal
MD (Pediatrics) DM (Neonatology)
Postgraduate Institute of Medical
Education and Research
Rohtak, Haryana, India

Kumar Ankur
MD (Pediatrics) DrNB (Neonatology)
BLK Max Superspeciality Hospital
New Delhi, India

Lalan Bharti MD (Pediatrics)
Jag Pravesh Chandra Hospital
New Delhi, India

Mahender Jain
MD (Pediatrics) DM (Neonatology)
All India Institute of Medical Sciences
Bhopal, Madhya Pradesh, India

Mangala Bharathi
MD (Pediatrics) DM (Neonatology)
Madras Medical College
Chennai, Tamil Nadu, India

Manoj Modi
MD (Pediatrics) DrNB (Neonatology)
Sir Ganga Ram Hospital
New Delhi, India

Manoj VC
MD (Pediatrics)
Jubilee Mission Medical College
and Research Institute
Thrissur, Kerala, India

Mohit Sahni MD (Pediatrics)
DCH DNB (Pediatrics) PDDNFU PDDPM
Nirmal Hospital
Surat, Gujarat, India

Monika Kaushal
MD (Pediatrics) DM (Neonatology)
Emirates Specialty Hospital
Dubai, UAE

Nalinikanta Panigrahi
MD (Pediatrics) DrNB (Neonatology)
Rainbow Children's Hospital
Hyderabad, Telangana, India

Naveen Gupta
MD (Pediatrics) DrNB (Neonatology)
Rainbow Children's Hospital
New Delhi, India

Nishad Plakkal
MD (Pediatrics)
Jawaharlal Institute of Postgraduate
Medical Education and Research
Puducherry, India
Residency in Neonatal-Perinatal
Medicine
Fellowship in Neonatal-Perinatal
Medicine

Pankaj Garg
MD (Pediatrics) DrNB (Neonatology)
Sir Ganga Ram Hospital
New Delhi, India

Parminder Singh Rooprai
MD (Pediatrics) DM Neonatology Fellow
All India Institute of Medical Sciences
New Delhi, India

Pradeep Debata
MD (Pediatrics) DM (Neonatology)
Vardhman Mahavir Medical College
and Safdarjung Hospital
New Delhi, India

Prashantha YN
MD (Pediatrics) DM (Neonatology)
Bangalore Baptist Hospital
Bengaluru, Karnataka, India

Pratima Anand
MD (Pediatrics) DM (Neonatology)
Lady Hardinge Medical College
and Associated Hospitals
New Delhi, India
National Co-ordinator, NEOMAP

Priyanka Gupta
MD (Pediatrics) DnRB (Neonatology)
Nutema Hospital
Meerut, Uttar Pradesh, India

Rajesh Kumar
MD (Pediatrics) DM (Neonatology)
Rani Hospital
Ranchi, Jharkhand, India

Ravi Sachan
MD (Pediatrics)
University College of Medical Sciences
New Delhi, India

Rishikesh Thakre
MD (Pediatrics) DM (Neonatology)
Neoclinic Hospital
Aurangabad, Maharashtra, India

Sameer Sheikh
MD (Pediatrics) DM (Neonatology)
Wockhardt Hospital
Mumbai, Maharashtra, India

Sandeep Kadam
MD (Pediatrics) DM (Neonatology)
BJ Government Medical College
Pune, Maharashtra, India

Sanjay Wazir
MD (Pediatrics) DM (Neonatology)
Motherhood Hospital
Gurugram, Haryana, India

Sindhu S
MD (Pediatrics) DM (Neonatology)
Kauveri Hospital
Chennai, Tamil Nadu, India

Somashekhar Nimbalkar
MD (Pediatrics)
Pramukhswami Medical College
Anand, Gujarat, India

Srinivas Murki
MD (Pediatrics) DM (Neonatology)
Paramitha Hospital
Hyderabad, Telangana, India

Suman Rao
MD (Pediatrics) DM (Neonatology)
St John's Hospital
Bengaluru, Karnataka, India

Surender Singh Bisht
MD (Pediatrics) DNB (Pediatrics)
Head and Senior Specialist
Department of Pediatrics
Swami Dayanand Hospital
New Delhi, India

Sushma Nangia
MD (Pediatrics) DM (Neonatology-AIIMS)
Director – Professor and Head
Department of Neonatology
Lady Hardinge Medical College and
Associated Kalawati Saran
Children Hospital
New Delhi, India

Tanushree Sahoo
MD (Pediatrics) DM (Neonatology)
All India Institute of Medical Sciences
Bhubaneswar, Odisha, India

Tejo Pratap Oleti
MD (Pediatrics) DM (Neonatology)
Fernandez Hospital
Hyderabad, Telangana, India

Usha Devi Rajendran
MD (Pediatrics) DNB (Pediatrics) DM
(Neonatology) DNB (Neonatology)
Jawaharlal Institute of Postgraduate
Medical Education and Research
Puducherry, India

Vijayanand Jamalpuri
MD (Pediatrics) MRCPH FRCPCH CCT Pediatrics
UK Fellowship in Neonatology, New Zealand
Rainbow Children's Hospital
Hyderabad, Telangana, India

Foreword

India has added a lot of infrastructure for newborn care both in the public and private sectors. There has been tremendous augmentation of Special Newborn Care Units (SNCUs) at the district level. These have contributed to improved survival of newborns in the country. However as more and more small and sicker babies are being managed in these facilities, there has been an increasing felt need amongst the healthcare providers to augment their procedural skills and increase 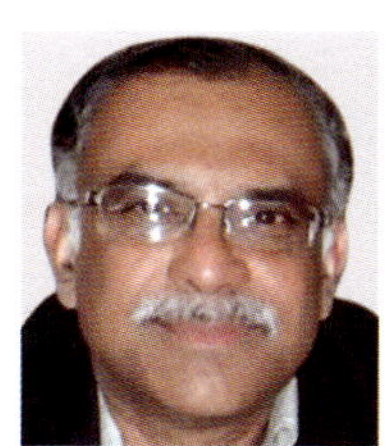 their knowledge regards the medications that are often required to be used for these babies. There is already a facility based newborn care (FBNC) training package that is being used by the government to train the staff at the SNCUs. The current training module on Neonatal Medication and Procedures (NEOMAP) is a complement to the existing SNCU training.

The current NEOMAP training program has identified 16 important procedural skills, and all of these are imparted entirely through hands on demonstration and practice on manikins that can simulate the clinical experience of the trainees. The program also covers several important medications that are needed for management of critically sick newborns and has a very important component of medication errors and is prevention. These modules have been refined based on feedback that was received during the initial pilot studies in different regions of the country and it is hoped that it will evolve and adapt with changing needs and practices.

The National Neonatology Forum (NNF) would like to place on record its gratitude to UNICEF for having supported the development of this program. We hope that the trainees who participate in this program will benefit in upgrading their skills for improving neonatal outcomes in the country at large and in their own facilities.

Siddharth Ramji
President
National Neonatology Forum (2022)

Foreword

National Neonatology Forum (NNF) of India established in 1980 has a mandate of improving the capacity and skills of neonatal healthcare providers in the country with a common goal of providing safe and effective quality care to every newborn.

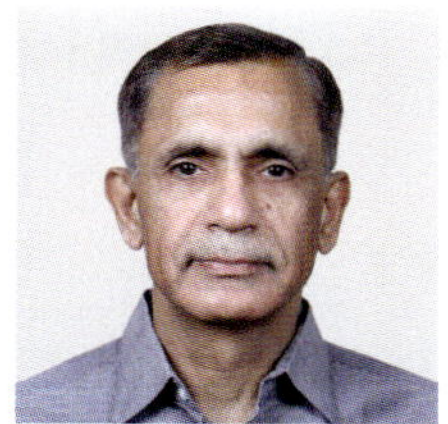

With advancements in technology and instrumentation suitable for newborns, the frequency of procedures and use of medications in the neonatal intensive care unit (NICU) has increased tremendously. Reportedly, a neonate in the NICU may undergo an average of 7–17 painful procedures per day. The preterm infants are exposed to these procedures with an even higher frequency. Though lifesaving, these procedures and medications have the potential of causing grave harm to the vulnerable neonate and negate all the potential benefits of these. It is a common observation that even simple and universal procedures such as intravenous cannula insertion, blood sampling, glucose monitoring, central line insertion, endotracheal intubation, suction, and surfactant administration are carried out with wide variability and often in an unsafe manner by healthcare providers. In fact, peripheral intravenous cannula is the single-most important source of healthcare-associated infections in our country. Similarly, the incidence of medication errors in NICUs is high with little awareness and efforts to improve the systems.

With the goal of enhancing the skills of our healthcare providers in providing medications and necessary procedures safely with minimum variability, the NNF launched Neonatal Medications and Procedures (NEOMAP) training module with standard operating protocols for common neonatal procedures and of medications. A series of NEOMAP hands-on workshops were conducted across the country and the module was tested and refined in multiple iterative cycles. This compendium is the result of tremendous efforts by more than 45 neonatology and nursing experts from the country, and hundreds of participants of NEOMAP workshops who provided excellent feedback and inputs.

I am happy to see that the compendium is now available as a publication for a broader outreach. I sincerely hope this will help standardize and make neonatal practice safer. I congratulate the NNF team for this humongous effort.

Praveen Kumar
Professor
Division of Neonatology, Department of Pediatrics
Postgraduate Institute of Medical Education and Research
Chandigarh, India
President, National Neonatology Forum (NNF), 2023

Foreword

Dear Friends and Academicians,

Greetings from National Neonatology Forum of India!

NEOMAP is a prestigious program of Central NNF launched as a part of Presidential Action Plan 2022.

NEOMAP is an abbreviated name for *Neonatal Medications and Procedures.*

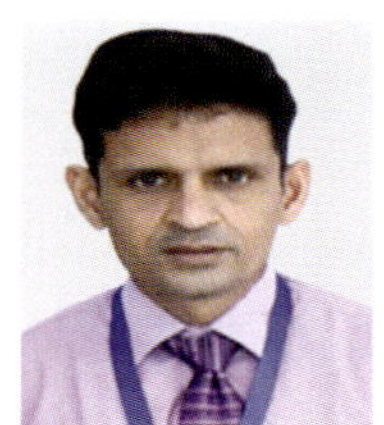

This program was launched as there was a felt need for a program where common neonatal procedures can be taught to delegates as hand on training in workstations. Also, medication errors are quite common in NICUs. To prevent this discussion about common drugs used in NICU and how to prevent medication errors was made a part of the program.

A formal proposal was sent to UNICEF to support the NEOMAP program which they readily agreed. Teams were formed to draw SOPs for common procedures and drugs and the whole program was designed and finalized in record time of 2 months. NNF office also procured mannequins for conducting these workstations.

The first NEOMAP program was held on 11th June 2022 in Kolkata, followed by programs in New Delhi and Varanasi. Looking at the popularity and demands, many states came forward to hold this program. Since then, about 10 programs have been organized in various states and zonal NEOCONs.

NNF is also organizing separate NEOMAP programs for doctors and nurses in NEOCON 2022.

We hope many more delegates are benefitted by this program. It also gives me immense pleasure to unveil the facilitators guide and workbook for NEOMAP in NEOCON 2022.

Long live NNF!!

Dinesh Tomar
Honorary Secretary
National Neonatology Forum (NNF)

Preface

Neonatal care is all about precision and accuracy. Even a small deviation in the provision of care can lead to magnified errors. Administration of medications and procedures are the most common skills needed for neonatal healthcare providers. Since administration of medications is one of the most common procedures and neonates are especially prone to adverse effects in case of errors, this manual hence incorporates Medications and Procedures together and called *NEOMAP (NEOnatal Medications and Procedures)*.

The NEOMAP manual includes two sections—the first section on "Medications", which covers neonate specific one pager on common categories of medications (emergency medications, sedation and analgesia, antimicrobials, antiepileptics, steroids, and medications for the use of cardiovascular neonatal illnesses). It has been taken care that postnatal day and gestation-specific doses are mentioned. This manual is one of the few which caters specifically to the neonatal dosages.

The second section is on "Procedures" and includes 24 common neonatal intensive care procedures, including central line placement, chest tube insertion, prevention of ventilator-associated pneumonia (VAP), and central line-associated bloodstream infection (CLABSI). The manual would be useful for all the healthcare providers involved in direct management of neonates. It includes nursing staff, medical officers working in special newborn care unit (SNCU), residents, and fellows in neonatology.

The coordinators are indebted to the contributing neonatology experts from all over the country, for their outstanding efforts in providing technical inputs for this manual. The experts of international repute have a total combined experience of managing more than a lakh neonate, and we have included many practical tips for the neonatal procedures.

We would like to express our appreciation to team UNICEF India office for the ongoing support for improving neonatal care through various initiatives and collaborations.

This manual is also a resource material for the NEOMAP training program conducted over one day and trained more than 250 neonatal care providers. The program also enabled NNF India to procure high-quality neonatology simulators, for the first time, for the demonstration of common intensive care neonatal procedures. The other resource material from this program in the form of pretest, post-test, Objective Structured Clinical Examination (OSCE) evaluation sheets, and workstation checklists, provided in the facilitators' manual, can be utilized for further training by the master trainers at their respective neonatal care units.

We hope that this contribution would serve its small part in improving the neonatal care in the country.

Amit Upadhyay
Pratima Anand

Acknowledgments

The editors would like to acknowledge all the learned faculties involved in making of this book. It was an arduous task of writing evidence-based procedures in detail, yet in a very simplified way. The reviewers did a painstaking job of customizing the procedures being useful to residents and consultants in all levels of neonatal care. Their vast experience of years of clinical practice was distinctly evident. Without their expertise and promptness, this book would have never become a reality.

We would like to thank the invaluable contribution of all the reviewers who customized and updated the write-ups that led to further improvement in quality, coherence, and content presentation of chapters.

This book would not have been possible without the inspiration of our teachers and mentors. Professor Ashok Deorari (President, NNF 2020) inspired us to know the nitty gritty of all procedures during our in-training days. Most of our clinical expertise today can be attributed to his training. This can be said for not just us but most of the authors and reviewers of the book. Dr Ranjan Kumar Pejaver (President, NNF 2021) was the one who conceptualized the exercise of taking the expertise of these procedures to the periphery, to all practitioners, resident doctors, nursing staff working in SNCUs, medical colleges, and small and big neonatal intensive care units across the country. This book may not have been possible without his vision.

Based on this manual, more than 50 workshops were conducted, and more than 500 nurses and doctors across India were trained. With each workshop and feedback of the trainers, the standard operating procedures (SOPs) were refined further, which finally culminated into the current form of this book. Professor Siddharth Ramji (President, NNF 2022) and Professor Praveen Kumar (President, NNF 2023) helped and guided all authors and reviewers in the final write-up of the book and provided valuable inputs in giving the book its present colors and content. Professor Sushma Nangia (President, NNF 2024) guided and supervised the final stages of book formatting and printing. The acknowledgement would be incomplete without thanking the NNF Secretaries (2021 to 2024, Dr Dinesh Tomar and Dr Surender Singh Bisht) for their active collaboration at all stages of this process.

We appreciate and acknowledge the contribution by the team of preterm care package-eliminating retinopathy of prematurity (ROP), for their support in formulation of assessments through multiple choice questions in NEOMAP and SOPs of few neonatal procedures (mentioned at the end of respective chapters as further reading, *https://www.pretermcare-eliminatingrop.com*).

Thank You

Amit Upadhyay
Pratima Anand

Contents

NNF NEOMAP Facilitators' Guide

◼ ABOUT NEOMAP

NEOMAP is based on the "Learn, See, Practice, Prove, Do, and Maintain" (LSPPDM) pedagogy and is one of the frameworks synthesized after intensely reviewing the literature, which is an evidence-based teaching and learning of procedural skills **(Fig. 1)**. This pedagogy uses cognitive and psychomotor domains of learning.

It exposes the learners in two phases: One is cognitive, and the other is psychomotor. In the cognitive phase, the learner meets the two steps of "Learn" and "See". The first step "Learn" is focusing on acquainting knowledge through online sharing of resources and pre-workshop assessment. Whereas the psychomotor phase deals with the steps of "Practice", "Prove", "Do", and "Maintain". In the "Practice" step learners deliberately perform the learned skill in the simulation environment. In the fourth step "Prove" the learner's skill was assessed on a simulator to prove proficiency. The fifth phase "DO", and sixth phase "Maintain" should be done under supervision in clinical scenarios till the trainee attains the competency of an expert".

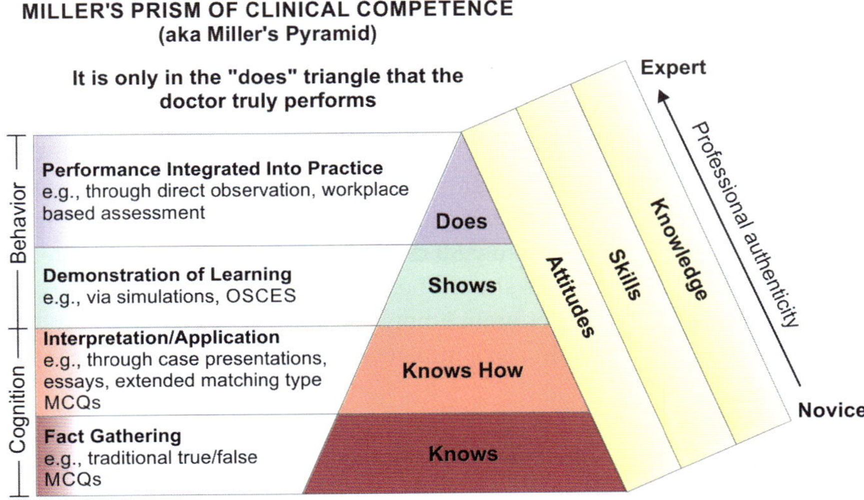

Fig. 1: The Millers pyramid explains the assessment of competence through MCQs and OSCEs and direct observations which are a part of NEOMAP.

Organizers and Coordinators

The educational module NEOMAP has to be conducted under the aegis of National Neonatology Forum (NNF), India, and United Nations Children's Fund, in collaborations with the respective state branches of NNF.

The team should consist of:
Target participants for NEOMAP: All the healthcare providers involved in direct management of neonates should undergo this skill-based training. It includes nursing staff, medical officers working in SNCUs, residents, and fellows in neonatology.

Facilitators: NEOMAP aims to enroll 32–36 participants per workshop and minimum 8 facilitators are needed. To standardize the key messages and demonstration of procedure in a uniform way across country, a workbook with standard operating procedures (SOP) for each procedure will be provided to the faculty at least 2 weeks prior to the workshop. Relevant video resources shall also be shared.

A team meeting 2 days prior to the workshop should be conducted to appraise the faculty about the intended content and time management of the workstations.

Teaching Mode and Methods

NEOMAP should incorporate the principle of adult teaching. It will be a blended learning with delegates expected to read through the standardized SOPs provided in the workbook along with video resources, combined with offline demonstration of skills on simulators in presence of the expert facilitators.

Venue of the Workshop

The venue can be decided based on consensus between the state and central NNF team. The venue can be a medical college, or a place reserved especially for the workshop. The venue should have the capacity to incorporate four workstations (with approximately 50 delegates and faculty) each at least 6–8 feet apart. The organizers should be cognizant that sufficient space is provided to avoid noise interference between the two stations, since it is interactive skill-based learning on simulators.

▪ ABOUT THE PROGRAM OF THE DAY

NEOMAP aims to impart skills through a 1-day workshop. (Template program is on next page)

- *Registration followed by introductory session:* Introduction of faculty and participants. Introduction to the workshop and its objectives in brief.
- *Division of participants groups:* Based on the composition of the cohort, the participants shall be divided into four groups of 8–10 each, who shall be rotating through four stations over 4 hours.
- Each workstation would be from 50 minutes to 1 hour. Since the delegates would have read through the content before attending the workshop, it is desirable that the facilitator invites two participants each to directly demonstrate the procedure strictly based on the checklist. Facilitator should enable them to do it themselves, correcting in between whenever the skill depicted in deviating from the checklist.
- *Tea and lunch:* Tea break after two rotations and lunch after completing the four stations.
- *Post-Lunch session:* Large group teaching on medications and prevention of medications
- Objective Structured Clinical Examination (OSCE) assessment over 90 minutes followed by post-test.

	• OSCE 1 • Endotracheal intubation • *(2 intubation heads, 2 simulator manikins, and other relevant consumables)*	• OSCE 2 • Intravenous (IV) cannulation • *(2 IV arms, 2 simulator manikins, and other relevant consumables)*	• OSCE 3 • Hand hygiene • *(4 bottles of hand rub)*
Group 1			
Group 2			
Group 3			
Group 4			

- Total time
- Elicitation ceremony and certificate distribution, followed by feedback session (verbal and written)

NEOMAP
TIME: 9.00 am to 4.45 pm
36 participants (4 groups)

Time	Topic
08.30 am to 09.00 am	Registration and Pre-Test
09.00 am to 09.10 am	Welcome, Inauguration, and Introduction to the program
09.10 am to 09.25 am	Role of skills in neonatal care
09.25 am to 09.30 am	Introduction to procedures module and division into Workgroups
4 Workstations (50 minutes each) 09.30 am to 1.30 pm 09.30 am to 10.20 am: Rotation 1 10.25 am to 11.15 am: Rotation 2 **11.15 am to 11.35 am: Tea** 11.35 am to 12.25 pm: Rotation 3 12.30 pm to 1.20 pm: Rotation 4	
Workstation 1	Venipuncture (blood sampling, blood culture, and dextrose monitoring), intravenous cannulation, SpO_2 and NIBP (noninvasive blood pressure) monitoring, and oro-/nasogastric tube insertion
Workstation 2	Central lines, PICC (peripherally inserted central catheter) line, CLABSI (central line-associated bloodstream infection) bundle
Workstation 3	Endotracheal (ET) intubation, ET suction, surfactant therapy ventilator-associated pneumonia (VAP) prevention bundle
Workstation 4	Hand hygiene, lumbar puncture, and exchange transfusion
1.25 pm to 2.15 pm: Lunch	
2.15 pm to 2.30 pm: Introduction to medication module	
2.30 pm to 3.00 pm: Minimizing medication errors	
3.00 pm to 4.30 pm: OSCE (3 procedures, 36 participants, 10 faculty) and Post-test OSCE stations on 1. Endotracheal intubation; 2. Intravenous cannulation; 3. Hand hygiene	
4.30 pm to 4.35 pm: Closing remarks: NNF team	
4.35 pm to 4.45 pm: Certificate distribution	

■ CONTENT OF WORKBOOK AND KEY MESSAGES

The workbook has two sections: (1) Common neonatal medications and (2) SOP for common neonatal procedures.

The SOP for each procedure is aimed at proving standardized information across all the workshops, even though it may be facilitated by different faculty experts.

The SOPs are a compilation of evidence-based, peer-reviewed resources and the same has been mentioned as suggested reading section. The compilation is an effort of more than 40 national experts in neonatology.

Common Key Messages on Each Station

- Asepsis, hand hygiene, and developmentally supportive care should be emphasized on each station before each procedure.
- Skin antisepsis should be as per the respective unit protocol (3 spirit swabs/chlorhexidine swabs/spirit/betadine/spirit swabs)
- Biomedical waste disposal (color of bags) may differ slightly in different units and should be followed as per the respective hospital infection control policy.
- Use of gloves for each procedure should be as per World Health Organization (WHO) policy **(Fig. 2)**.

This workbook should be provided to the participants at least 2 weeks before the scheduled workshop followed by the MCQ-based assessment (before the workshop), so that participants come prepared and have adequate time to practice on simulator on the day of workshop.

Though the workbook contains an additional one pager on medications and a few other procedures, the workshop will cover the following procedures, as already described in the program section.

- Lumbar puncture
- Exchange transfusion
- Hand hygiene
- Orogastric (OG) tube insertion
- Dextrose monitoring
- IV cannulation
- Venipuncture and blood sampling
- Blood culture
- SpO_2 monitoring
- NIBP monitoring
- Umbilical artery catheter (UAC) and umbilical venous catheter (UVC) insertion
- PICC line insertion
- Endotracheal intubation
- Endotracheal suction

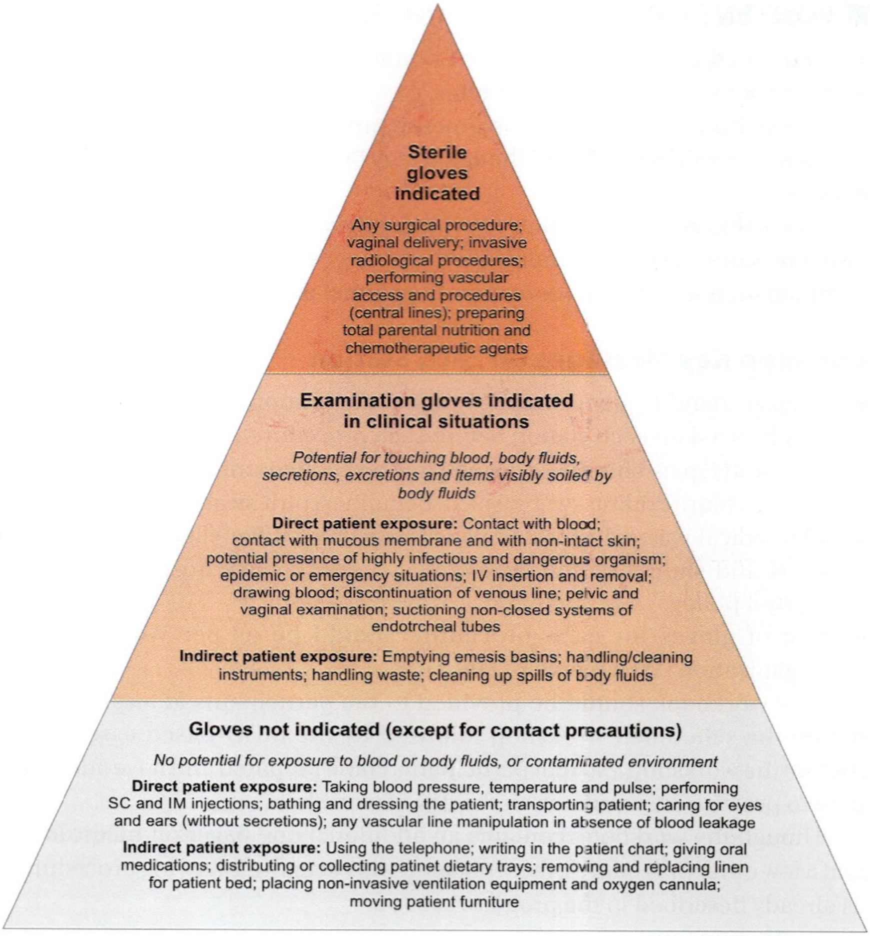

Fig. 2: Guide to use of gloves for common clinical procedures.

- Surfactant administration
- Prevention of VAP and CLABSI.

ROLES AND RESPONSIBILITIES FOR ORGANIZING THE WORKSHOP

Role of the Central Coordinating Team (NNF India)

- Provision of manikins
- Allocation of stipulated budget
- Two national faculty for the workshop
- Coordinating with the regional organizers
- Provision of blended teaching through online resources (videos and soft copy of workbook) and offline OSCE, pre-test, post-test, and feedback.

Role of the Regional Organizers

- Coordination with the central team
- Identification of participants and creating of online group for dissemination of resources at least 2 weeks prior to scheduled workshop
- Identification of at least six regional faculty for workshop
- Venue arrangement
- Arrangement of consumables for each workstation (Checklist provided ahead)
- Other logistics for registration and felicitation/certification.

■ CHECKLISTS FOR THE WORKSTATIONS

Manikins (Central NNF)

- Four simulator manikins (for venipuncture, exchange transfusion, and UAC/UVC insertion)
- Two intravenous arms (PICC line and blood culture)
- One lumbar puncture manikin
- Two central lines [internal jugular vein (IJV) and femoral insertion]
- Two intubation heads.

Consumables and Disposables (Regional Organizers)

General Checklist

1. Instructor folder with: (i) program copy, (ii) pen, (iii) notebook, and (iv) manual printout
2. Participant folder: Same things
3. Four workstation tables
4. Badges for participants and faculty
5. One basic banner
6. Attendance sheet for participants and faculty
7. OSCE printouts
8. Pretest and post-test printouts
9. Audiovisual media
10. Water and food
11. Workstation labels 1–4 and OSCEs labels 1–3
12. Feedback sheets printouts
13. Certificates

Checklist for Workstation 1
[Venipuncture (for all sampling), intravenous cannulation, SpO_2 and NIBP monitoring, and oro-/nasogastric tube insertion]

1. Intravenous arm simulator
2. Basic Manikins for OG tube insertion, pulse oximetry probe fixation
3. Gloves

4. Sterillium
5. Sampling needles
6. 1 mL, 2 mL, and 5 mL syringes
7. Blood culture bottles
8. Spirit swabs/chlorhexidine swabs
9. Neopore/micropore/tegaderm
10. OG tube 5–8 FG
11. Stethoscope
12. 5-mL syringe
13. Dummy feed
14. Pulse oximeter
15. BP cuff, BP instrument, and multipara monitor
16. IV cannulation manikin
17. Glucometer with strips

*Checklist for Workstation 2**
(Central lines, PICC line, and CLABSI bundle)
1. Intravenous arm for PICC line
2. Manikin with umbilical cord for umbilical vessel catheterization
3. Central line insertion manikin (for IJV and femoral catheterization)
4. Leaderflex newborn sizes
5. PICC lines (premicath) 24–28 F sizes (2 in number)
6. USG machine with linear probe
7. Gloves
8. Sterillium
9. Donning and doffing gowns, cap, and mask (4 in number)
10. Spirit and betadine swabs for skin preparation
11. Forceps to hold the UAC/UVC
12. Umbilical catheters (newborn sizes: 3.0, 3.5, 4.0, and 5.0)

*Checklist for Workstation 3**
(Endotracheal intubation, ET suction, and surfactant therapy VAP prevention bundle)
1. Intubation heads (2)
2. ET size 2.5–3.5
3. Laryngoscope with blades (2 in number) with extra batteries
4. Stethoscope
5. Leucoplast, Tegaderm, and micropore for fixation
6. Ambu bag and mask
7. Suction catheters size 6–10
8. Gloves
9. Sterillium
10. Surfactant bottle
11. OG tubes 5–8 FG

12. Blade
13. Sterile tray and spirit and betadine swabs
14. Pulse oximeter
15. Surfcath for LISA demonstration
16. CPAP/circuits, if possible, for VAP prevention bundle

*Checklist for Workstation 4**
(Hand Hygiene, Lumbar Puncture, and Exchange Transfusion)
1. LP manikin
2. Manikin with umbilical cord for exchange transfusion
3. Sterillium/hand rub
4. Basic manikin
5. Three-way stop clocks (4 in number)
6. IV fluid connectors
7. Discarding bottle
8. Blood transfusion set
9. Umbilical catheters from 5–8 size
10. Syringes 1 mL, 2 mL, 5 mL, and 10 mL
11. Normal saline
12. Ambu bag
13. Pulse oximeter
14. Exchange transfusion monitoring checklist
15. Donning gowns, cap, and mask (3 each)
16. Sterile tray
17. Spirit and betadine swabs
18. Cord tie for umbilical cord insertion

Medications

- Emergency Medications
- Medications for Cardiovascular System
- Steroids
- Medications for Sedation and Analgesia
- Antimicrobials
- Antiepileptics
- Prevention of Medication Errors

Emergency Medications

Dobutamine

■ NAME OF THE DRUG (SUPPLIED AS)

Trade names: Dobutrex, Dobutam

■ INDICATIONS

- Sympathomimetic and inotropic agent
- Treatment of hypotension and hypoperfusion especially related to myocardial dysfunction.

■ PHARMACOKINETICS AND PHARMACODYNAMICS

- Synthetic catecholamine with mainly beta-1-adrenergic activity
- It is an inotrope and vasopressor.
- Increases myocardial contractility, cardiac index, oxygen delivery, and oxygen consumption.

■ AVAILABLE FORMULATIONS (SUPPLIED AS)

- Each vial contains 250 mg of lyophilized dobutamine hydrochloride.
- Also available as injection: 50 mg/mL

■ ROUTE

- Administer by intravenous (IV) or intraosseous (IO) route as a continuous infusion.
- Avoid bolus administration of the drug.
- Infusion into a large vein is preferred to minimize risk of tissue extravasation.

■ DOSE AND MAXIMUM DOSE (TOTAL DAILY DOSE)

Continuous IV infusion: 2–20 µg/kg/min; start at a low dose and titrate based on monitoring.

CAUTION, PRECAUTIONS, AND RED FLAGS (DRUG INTERACTIONS)

- Vials must be diluted prior to use in compatible diluent (D5W, D10W, NS) up to a concentration of 2000 µg/mL.
- Solutions containing dobutamine may exhibit a pink color due to oxidation of the drug. However, there is no significant loss of potency over 24 hours.
- Dobutamine infusion may cause hypotension if patient is hypovolemic. Therefore, assessment of volume status is must before starting infusion.
- Tachycardia and arrythmia can occur at high dosage.
- Prevent *Extravasation*
  - Central line administration is recommended to avoid extravasation.
  - Administer into a large vein to prevent extravasation; use an infusion device to control rates of flow.
  - Observe IV site frequently for signs of extravasation and/or infiltration.
  - Extravasation may cause tissue necrosis and sloughing of surrounding tissue and infiltration causes local inflammatory changes.
  - If extravasation is recognized, stop and disconnect the IV infusion but leave the catheter in place.
    - Antidote for extravasation is phentolamine: Inject a 0.5 mg/mL solution of phentolamine into the affected area. The usual amount needed is 1–5 mL, depending on the size of the infiltrate.

ADMINISTRATION AND EXAMPLE OF PRESCRIPTION (DILUTION)

- D5W, D10W, NS, dextrose–saline solutions, lactated Ringer's (LR)
- *Incompatible with alkaline solutions including sodium bicarbonate.

Example:

- Initiate dobutamine infusion at 10 µg/kg/min in a 1 kg neonate
- Dobutamine (mg) in 50-mL solution

    = 3 × body weight × (µg/kg/min)

    = 3 × 1 × 10

    = 30 mg

Dobutamine is available as 50 mg/1 mL in ampules. Dilute 1 mL in 9-mL NS to get 5 mg in 10 mL. Add 30 mg (6 mL with concentration 5 mg/mL) of Dobutamine to make up to 50 mL in an appropriate diluent (with 44 mL of NS) and infuse at the rate of 1 mL/h to provide 10 µg/kg/min.

CONTRAINDICATIONS

No specific contraindication; assess fluid status before starting infusion.

ADVERSE EFFECTS

- *Cardiovascular:* Ectopic heartbeats, tachycardia, elevation in blood pressure, at higher doses ventricular tachycardia or arrhythmias
- *Central nervous system (CNS):* Headache in children and adults
- *Gastrointestinal:* Nausea, vomiting
- *Local:* Phlebitis
- *Respiratory:* Dyspnea

MONITORING AND PREVENTION OF EXTRAVASATION (COMMENTS)

- Continuous heart rate [preferably using electrocardiogram (ECG)] and blood pressures (preferably invasive intra-arterial blood pressure) monitoring and urine output; monitor fluid balance and electrolytes.
- Tachyphylaxis (downregulation of beta receptors) to the hemodynamic effect may occur over time, especially in neonates. Therefore, alternate inotropes may need to be considered.
- Relative adrenal insufficiency, especially in premature neonates and infants with perinatal asphyxia, may be the underlying cause of hypotension. Administration of hydrocortisone may be required in such scenarios.
- Do not flush line to check patency.

FURTHER READING

1. Dempsey E, Rabe H. The Use of Cardiotonic Drugs in Neonates. Clin Perinatol. 2019;46(2):273-90.
2. Gupta S, Donn SM. Neonatal hypotension: dopamine or dobutamine? Semin Fetal Neonatal Med. 2014;19(1):54-9.

Dopamine

■ NAME OF THE DRUG (SUPPLIED AS)

Trade names: Domin, Dopar, Dopress, Dopacin

■ INDICATIONS

- Sympathomimetic and inotropic agent
- Used for treatment of hypotension.

■ PHARMACOKINETICS AND PHARMACODYNAMICS

- Dopamine is a naturally occurring precursor of noradrenaline. It acts on dopaminergic, alpha- and beta-adrenergic receptors.
- *Low dose (0.5–2 µg/kg/min):* Dopaminergic effects predominate vasodilator effects in the renal, coronary, mesenteric, and cerebral vascular beds.
- *Higher dose (>5 µg/kg/min):* Alpha- and beta-adrenergic effects cause inotropic, chronotropic, and peripheral vasoconstrictor effects.
- In neonates, the effects of varied dose of dopamine on various receptors is uncertain due to developmental differences in endogenous norepinephrine stores, alpha- and beta-adrenergic, and dopamine receptor functions, and myocardial function.

■ AVAILABLE FORMULATIONS (SUPPLIED AS)

Available as 200 mg/5 mL ampules

■ ROUTE

- Administer by intravenous (IV) or intraosseous (IO) route as a continuous infusion.
- Avoid bolus administration of the drug.
- Infusion into a large vein is preferred to minimize risk of tissue extravasation.

■ DOSE AND MAXIMUM DOSE

- *Continuous IV infusion:* 2–20 µg/kg/min
- Start at a low dose and titrate based on monitoring.

■ CAUTION, PRECAUTIONS, AND RED FLAGS (COMMENTS)

- Vials must be diluted prior to use in compatible diluent [D5W, D10W, NS (normal saline)] up to a concentration of 1,600 µg/mL.
- Diluted solutions stable for 24 hours; do not use if color change is noted.

- Tachycardia and arrythmia can occur at high dosage.
- *Prevent extravasation using same rules that stated for dobutamine.*

ADMINISTRATION AND EXAMPLE OF PRESCRIPTION (DILUTION)

- D5W, D10W, NS, dextrose–saline solutions, LR (lactated Ringer's)
- *Incompatible with alkaline solutions including sodium bicarbonate

Example:
Initiate dopamine infusion at 10 µg/kg/min in a 1 kg neonate

Dopamine (mg) in 50 mL solution
$$= 3 \times \text{body weight} \times (\mu g/kg/min)$$
$$= 3 \times 1 \times 10$$
$$= 30 \text{ mg}$$

Dopamine is available as 40 mg/1 mL in ampules. Dilute 1 mL in 9-mL normal saline to get 4 mg in 10 mL. Add 30 mg (7.5 mL with concentration 4 mg/mL) of dobutamine to make up to 50 mL in an appropriate diluent (with 42.5 mL of normal saline) and infuse at the rate of 1 mL/h to provide 10 µg/kg/min.

CONTRAINDICATIONS

No specific contraindication; assess fluid status before starting infusion.

ADVERSE EFFECTS

- Tachycardia and arrythmia
- *Local:* Phlebitis

MONITORING (COMMENTS)

- Continuous heart rate [preferably using ECG (electrocardiogram)] and blood pressures (preferably invasive intra-arterial blood pressure) monitoring and urine output; monitor fluid balance and electrolytes.
- Do not flush line to check patency.

FURTHER READING

1. Dempsey E, Rabe H. The Use of Cardiotonic Drugs in Neonates. Clin Perinatol. 2019;46(2):273-90.
2. Gupta S, Donn SM. Neonatal hypotension: dopamine or dobutamine? Semin Fetal Neonatal Med. 2014;19(1):54-9.

Adrenaline or Epinephrine

■ NAME OF THE DRUG (SUPPLIED AS)

Trade names: Vasocon, Adrenaline

■ INDICATIONS

Sympathomimetic and inotropic agent

■ PHARMACOKINETICS AND PHARMACODYNAMICS

Epinephrine (adrenaline) is the major hormone secreted by the adrenal medulla.

It is a potent stimulator of all four adrenergic receptors ($\alpha1$, $\alpha2$, $\beta1$, and $\beta2$).

Effects of epinephrine in the body depend on the dose of epinephrine, number of receptors available on target tissues, and the affinity of these receptors

Action on α_1 receptors leads to peripheral vasoconstriction.

Action on $\beta1$ receptors in the myocardium leads to chronotropy (increased heart rate), inotropy (increased contractility), dromotropy (increase conduction velocity), and lusitropy (increased rate of myocardial relaxation).

Stimulation of α_2 receptors leads to presynaptic inhibition of norepinephrine release in the CNS and vasoconstriction of coronary arteries.

Through $\beta2$ receptor stimulation, it causes vascular smooth muscle relaxation and increased myocardial contractility. This $\beta2$ receptor-mediated coronary vasodilation may contribute to improved coronary perfusion following epinephrine administration during cardiopulmonary resuscitation.

■ AVAILABLE FORMULATIONS (SUPPLIED AS AND DOSE)

- Epinephrine is available as a sterile solution for injection in the following concentrations and sizes: 1:1,000 (1 mg/mL) solution in 1 mL preservative-free ampoules.
- All epinephrine products should be stored at room temperature and protected from freezing and excessive heat and light.
- Do not use the injection, if it contains a precipitate or is pinkish or darker than slightly yellow.
- Dilutions for infusion should be prepared every 24 hours and protected from light by covering the IV infusion with an amber bag.

Note: 1:10,000 = 0.1 mg/mL and 1:1,000 = 1 mg/mL

■ ROUTE

- IV (preferably umbilical vein), intraosseous, or endotracheal (ET) for resuscitation
- IV for continuous infusion

■ DOSE AND MAXIMUM DOSE

Resuscitation:

- IV dose is 0.01–0.03 mg/kg, followed by a normal saline (NS) flush.
- If umbilical venous access has not yet been obtained, epinephrine may be given by the ET route in a dose of 0.05–0.1 mg/kg. The dosage can be repeated every 3–5 minutes. Follow ET administration with several positive pressure ventilations.
- Do not administer these higher doses of epinephrine intravenously.
  IV continuous infusion: Start at 0.1 µg/kg/min and adjust to desired response, to a maximum of 1 µg/kg/.

Shock: IV 0.05–0.3 µg/kg/min; range 0.05–1 µg/kg/min

Example:

- Initiate Adrenaline infusion at 0.3 µg/kg/min in a 1 kg neonate
- Adrenaline (mg) in 50 mL solution

  $$= 3 \times \text{body weight} \times (\text{µg/kg/min})$$
  $$= 3 \times 1 \times 1$$
  $$= 3 \text{ mg}$$

- Add 3 mg of adrenaline (3 mL of adrenaline with 1 mg/mL concentration) to make up to 50 mL in an appropriate dilution (with 47 mL of NS) and infuse at the rate of 0.3 mL/h (note that 1 mL/h will provide 1 µg/kg/min of Adrenaline)

■ CAUTION, PRECAUTIONS, AND RED FLAGS (COMMENTS)

- Epinephrine should be stored at room temperature and protected from freezing, excessive heat, and light. It is light-sensitive.
- Dilutions for infusion should be prepared every 24 hours and protected from light by covering with a brown bag.
- *Follow rules to avoid extravasation like dobutamine.*

■ ADMINISTRATION AND EXAMPLE OF PRESCRIPTION (COMPATIBILITY)

- D5W, D10W, and NS; although NS is compatible, administration in saline solution alone is not recommended.
- Dextrose protects against oxidation of epinephrine.

■ CONTRAINDICATIONS

No specific contraindication

■ ADVERSE EFFECTS

- *Cardiovascular:* Cardiac arrhythmias, tachycardia, hypertension, pallor
- *Gastrointestinal:* Nausea, vomiting
- *Metabolic:* Transient elevation of blood sugar, hypokalemia, lactic acidosis
- *Renal:* Decreased renal and splanchnic blood flow

■ MONITORING AND PRECAUTIONS (COMMENTS)

- Monitor electrocardiogram (ECG), blood pressure, heart rate, respiratory rate, oxygenation, neurological status, and fluid balance.
- Excessive increases in blood pressure may occur in patients receiving doses >0.3 µg/kg/min.
- Monitor blood glucose (hyperglycemia is an expected outcome) and serum potassium.

■ FURTHER READING

1. Dempsey E, Rabe H. The Use of Cardiotonic Drugs in Neonates. Clin Perinatol. 2019;46(2):273-90.
2. Noori S, Seri I. Neonatal blood pressure support: the use of inotropes, lusitropes, and other vasopressor agents. Clin Perinatol. 2012;39(1):221-38.

Noradrenaline or Norepinephrine

■ NAME OF THE DRUG

Trade names: Norad, N-Adrin, Adrenor

■ INDICATIONS

Sympathomimetic and inotropic agent

■ PHARMACOKINETICS AND PHARMACODYNAMICS

Norepinephrine, a sympathomimetic amine, has both alpha-adrenergic activity, resulting in peripheral vasoconstriction, and beta-adrenergic activity leading to inotropic stimulation of the heart and coronary artery vasodilation.

■ AVAILABLE FORMULATIONS

4 mg/2 mL ampules

■ ROUTE

- Preferred route is venous.
- Intraosseous route is an option but is not preferred especially for preterm newborns.

■ DOSE AND MAXIMUM DOSE

- Initial dose, 0.2–0.5 µg/kg/min by intravenous (IV) infusion
- Titrate every 30 minutes to target blood pressure.
- Usual infusion rate 0.2–2 µg/kg/min; higher rates may be required.

■ CAUTION, PRECAUTIONS, AND RED FLAGS

- Hypovolemia should be corrected prior to initiating norepinephrine.
- Monitor blood pressure, heart rate, urine output, and peripheral perfusion.
- Assess extremities for changes in color or temperature.
- *Follow rules to avoid extravasation like dobutamine*

■ ADMINISTRATION AND EXAMPLE OF PRESCRIPTION

D5W, D5NS, normal saline (NS), lactated Ringer's (LR)

Example:
- Initiate noradrenaline infusion at 1 µg/kg/min in a 1 kg neonate

- Noradrenaline (mg) in 50-mL solution
    = 3 × body weight × (μg/kg/min)
    = 3 × 1 × 1
    = 3 mg
- Add 3 mg of noradrenaline (1.5 mL of nor adrenaline with 2 mg/mL concentration) to make up to 50 mL in an appropriate dilution (with 48.5 mL of NS) and infuse at the rate of 1 mL/h (note that 1 mL/h will provide 1 μg/kg/min of noradrenaline)

CONTRAINDICATIONS

- Contraindicated in hypotension due to blood volume deficits (except in emergency until blood can be administered), mesenteric or peripheral vascular thrombosis, and in presence of profound hypoxia or hypercarbia symptoms
- Contains sodium metabisulfite, which may cause allergic-type reactions

ADVERSE EFFECTS

- *Cardiovascular:* Cardiac arrhythmias, tachycardia, hypertension, pallor
- *Gastrointestinal:* Nausea, vomiting
- *Metabolic:* Transient elevation of blood sugar, hypokalemia, lactic acidosis
- *Renal:* Decreased renal and splanchnic blood flow

MONITORING AND PRECAUTIONS

- Monitor electrocardiogram (ECG), blood pressure, heart rate, respiratory rate, oxygenation, neurological status, and fluid balance.
- Excessive increases in blood pressure may occur in patients receiving doses >0.3 μg/kg/min.
- Monitor blood glucose (hyperglycemia is an expected outcome) and serum potassium.

FURTHER READING

1. Dempsey E, Rabe H. The Use of Cardiotonic Drugs in Neonates. Clin Perinatol. 2019;46(2):273-90.
2. Noori S, Seri I. Neonatal blood pressure support: the use of inotropes, lusitropes, and other vasopressor agents. Clin Perinatol. 2012;39(1):221-38.

Vasopressin

■ NAME OF THE DRUG

Trade names: CPressin, Vasopin, Pressyn, Cevas-20

■ INDICATIONS

- Antidiuretic action (used in management of diabetes insipidus)
- Vasoconstrictor (used in hypovolemic shock and to control bleeding in esophageal varices)
- In neonates, it is used in refractory catecholamine-resistant hypotension.

■ PHARMACOKINETICS AND PHARMACODYNAMICS

- Vasopressin is antidiuretic hormone formed in the hypothalamus and secreted by the posterior pituitary.
- *It acts on three receptors:*
  1. V1 receptors are present in blood vessels and mediate vasoconstriction in the systemic, splanchnic, renal, and coronary circulation. Vasopressin has minimal to no inotropic or chronotropic effects, maintains cardiac function, and may cause pulmonary vasodilation. Its vasoconstrictive effects are preserved during hypoxia and severe acidosis.
  2. V2 are present in the kidneys and regulate water absorption through antidiuretic effect. Thus, increasing the blood volume, cardiac output, and arterial pressure.
  3. V3 regulates the effects on the CNS such as the release of the neurotransmitter adrenocorticotrophic hormone (ACTH).

■ AVAILABLE FORMULATIONS

Vasopressin injection is available as a 20 U/mL sterile colorless solution in 1-mL vials.

■ ROUTE

Continuous IV infusion

■ DOSE AND MAXIMUM DOSE

- Initial 0.0001–0.0003 U/kg/min
- Titrate as needed to a maximum rate of 0.008 U/kg/min
- Target based on increase in systemic arterial blood pressure without undue adverse effects

■ CAUTION, PRECAUTIONS, AND RED FLAGS

- Use caution when giving with the following associated conditions: seizure disorders, headache, asthma, heart problems, renal failure.
- Intact vials should be stored at room temperature and protected from freezing.
- Unused portions should be discarded after use.
- Diluted solutions in compatible intravenous (IV) fluids are stable for 24 hours at room temperature.
- Can cause tissue ischemia and necrosis; management of vasopressin extravasation includes:
  - Stopping vasopressor infusion
  - Elevating the affected limb
  - For high-risk extravasations, use intradermal phentolamine 5–10 mg mixed in 10-mL sterile saline injected into the affected area.

■ ADMINISTRATION AND EXAMPLE OF PRESCRIPTION

D5W, normal saline (NS), dextrose–saline combinations

Example:

For an infant of 1 kg for dose 0.0003 U/kg/min

Add 1 mL of 20 U/mL vasopressin in 49 mL NS to get 20 U/50 mL (equivalent to 0.4 U/mL). Take 25 mL of this and add 25 mL of NS to obtain vasopressin of 0.2 U/mL concentration.

Infusion dose in (U/kg/min) = 0.0003 × 1 × 60 = 0.018 U/h

Infusion rate (mL/h)	Dose in U/h	Dose in U/kg/min
0.1	0.02	0.0003
0.2	0.04	0.0006
0.5	0.1	0.001
1	0.2	0.003

Hence, infusion rate is set at 0.1 mL/h

■ CONTRAINDICATIONS

Vascular diseases

■ ADVERSE EFFECTS

- Adverse effects are infrequent at lower doses but increase in frequency at higher doses.
- Common: Circumoral pallor, sweating, tremor
- At higher dose, it may produce increased blood pressure, bradycardia, minor arrhythmias, heart block, peripheral vascular constriction, decreased cardiac output, and myocardial ischemia and infarction.
- Limb ischemia

■ MONITORING

- Electrocardiogram (ECG)—used to monitor the hormone's cardiac effects during IV therapy
- Observe for signs of fluid overload
- Monitor electrolytes.

■ FURTHER READING

1. Meyer S, Gortner L, McGuire W, Baghai A, Gottschling S. Vasopressin in catecholamine-refractory shock in children. Anaesthesia. 2008;63(3):228-34.
2. Ni M, Kaiser JR, Moffett BS, Rhee CJ, Placencia J, Dinh KL, et al. Use of vasopressin in neonatal intensive care unit patients with hypotension. J Pediatr Pharmacol Ther. 2017;22(6):430-5.

Medications for Cardiovascular System

Paracetamol

■ INDICATIONS

Fever/pain, closure of patent ductus arteriosus (PDA)

■ PHARMACOKINETICS AND PHARMACODYNAMICS

Half-life is around 3 hours in term neonates and 5–11 hours in preterm neonates. Elimination is prolonged liver dysfunction.

■ AVAILABLE FORMULATIONS

Oral solution 250 mg/5 mL, drops 100 mg/mL, intravenous (IV) (infusion: 1 mL contains 5 mg)

Ampoule should not be used as it contains benzyl alcohol.

■ PREPARATION

No further dilution required

■ ROUTE

Intravenous, oral, and per rectal

■ DOSE

For fever/pain:
- *Preterm <32 weeks*: 12–15 mg/kg/dose 12 hourly
- *Preterm >32 weeks*: 12–15 mg/kg/dose 8 hourly
- *Term*: 12–15 mg/kg/dose 6 hourly

For PDA closure:
- 15 mg/kg/dose IV or oral 6 hourly for 3–5 days
- Caution, precautions, and red flags
- Use with caution in hepatic disease

■ ADVERSE EFFECTS

Pain at injection site, vomiting, rash, fever

■ CONTRAINDICATION

Intravenous formulation is contraindicated in severe liver impairment.

■ FURTHER READING

1. Cuzzolin L, Antonucci R, Fanos V. Paracetamol (acetaminophen) efficacy and safety in the newborn. Curr Drug Metab. 2013;14:178-85.
2. Pacifici GM, Allegaert K. Clinical pharmacology of paracetamol in neonates: a review. Curr Ther Res Clin Exp. 2014;77:24-30.

Ibuprofen

■ INDICATION

Closure of patent ductus arteriosus (PDA)

■ PHARMACOKINETICS AND PHARMACODYNAMICS

Half-life is around 15–43 hours irrespective of gestational age. Oral formulation is well-absorbed in preterm neonates.

■ AVAILABLE FORMULATIONS

Oral solution 100 mg/5 mL

■ PREPARATION

No further dilution required.

■ ROUTE

Oral, IV preparation not available in India

■ DOSE

10 mg/kg/dose oral followed by 5 mg/kg/dose at 24 and 48 hours

■ CAUTION, PRECAUTIONS, AND RED FLAGS

Use with caution in hypertension, heart disease, liver disease, and renal injury

■ ADVERSE EFFECTS

Gastrointestinal (GI) bleed, acute kidney injury (AKI), rash, increase in bilirubin

■ CONTRAINDICATIONS

Neonates allergic to other nonsteroidal anti-inflammatory drugs (NSAIDs), AKI, bleeding neonate

■ FURTHER READING

1. Gummin DD, Mowry JB, Beuhler MC, Spyker DA, Brooks DE, Dibert KW, et al. 2019 Annual Report of the American Association of Poison Control Centers' National Poison Data System (NPDS): 37th Annual Report. Clin Toxicol (Phila). 2020;58:1360.
2. Drug Information for the Health Care Professional USPDI 19th edition. United States: Thomson Micromedex; 1999. p. 388.

Drugs Used for Persistent Pulmonary Hypertension Sildenafil

■ TRADE NAMES WITH CONCENTRATION

Oral Rivatio (20 mg), Viagra (25 mg, 50 mg, 100 mg), Suhagra (100 mg), sildenafil tablets from Manforce (50 mg), Pulmosil oral suspension (10 mL)

Injection: Revatio (10 mg/mL), Assurans 10 mg/12.5 mL

■ INDICATIONS

Sildenafil is used as an adjuvant therapy to inhale nitric oxide (iNO) in cases of refractory acute PPHN (persistent pulmonary hypertension). Where iNO is not available in resource-limited settings, it can be used as primary therapy.

■ PHARMACOKINETICS AND PHARMACODYNAMICS

- Neonates demonstrate higher clearance as well as higher volume of distribution resulting in fluctuation of sildenafil concentrations.
- Further clearance rate is dependent on gestational age (increases with gestation) and co-administration of other cytochrome P450 enzyme inhibitors (e.g., fluconazole, ciprofloxacin, erythromycin) might increase its toxicity

■ DOSE AND ROUTE

- Can be administered both intravenous (IV) and oral route
- *Continuous IV infusion:*
  - *Loading dose:* 0.4 mg/kg administered over 3 hours, to minimize the risk of hypotension
  - *Maintenance dose:* 0.067 mg/kg/h as continuous IV infusion for up to 7 days
- *Oral:* A wide range of dosage has been reported.
  - *Initial:* 0.5 mg/kg/dose Q8–12 hours
  - *Maximum dose:* 1–2 mg/kg/dose Q6 hourly (4 mg/kg/day)

■ CAUTION, PRECAUTIONS, RED FLAGS, AND MONITORING

- Caution should be executed with concurrent use of nitrates (nitroglycerine).
- In case of liver failure or renal insufficiency, there should be extra precautions.

■ CONTRAINDICATIONS

Hypotension and concurrent use of drugs, such as ciprofloxacin and erythromycin.

■ ADVERSE EFFECT

Acute use: Hypotension

■ TEMPLATE PRESCRIPTION WITH AN EXAMPLE

Intravenous route: Available in India as 0.8 mg/1-mL solution. For IV bolus @ 0.4 mg/kg over 3 hours for a 3 kg baby 1.5 mL of 0.8 mg/1 mL injection needs to be diluted in 4.5 mL of normal saline (to make final solution of 6 mL) and then to be infused @ 2 mL/h for 3 hours. For maintenance dose of 0.067 mg/kg/h for a 3 kg baby total dose of $0.067 \times 3 \times 24 = 4.8$ mg of IV sildenafil (6 mL of 0.8 mg/1 mL solution) should be diluted in 18 mL normal saline and infused @ 1mL/h.

Oral route: Syrup Pulmosil (10mL) is available in India.

It is also easily available in 20 mg, 25 mg, 50 mg, and 100 mg tablets, which can be divided, and sachets can be prepared as per requirement. They need to be dissolved in water or milk for administration.

■ FURTHER READING

1. Perez KM, Laughon M. Sildenafil in Term and Premature Infants: A Systematic Review. Clin Ther. 2015;37(11):2598-607.e1.
2. Shah PS, Ohlsson A. (2011). Sildenafil for pulmonary hypertension in neonates. Available from: https://www.cochranelibrary.com/cdsr/doi/10.1002/14651858.CD005494.pub3/full [Last accessed February, 2024].
3. Steinhorn RH, Kinsella JP, Pierce C, Butrous G, Dilleen M, Oakes M, et al. Intravenous Sildenafil in the Treatment of Neonates with Persistent Pulmonary Hypertension. J Pediatr. 2009;155(6):841-7.e1.

Milrinone

■ TRADE NAMES/FORMULATION

Injectible salt milrinone lactate, commonly available brands with concentration: Primacor, Milvas, Milor, Milrineon 10 mg/10 mL.

■ INDICATIONS

- Milrinone is used as prophylaxis in low cardiac output states as prophylaxis in postcardiac surgery in neonates.
- Persistent pulmonary hypertension (PPHN) along with signs of left ventricular failure, especially as an adjuvant to inhaled nitric oxide (iNO) in cases of refractory PPHN (low level of evidence).

■ PHARMACOKINETICS AND PHARMACODYNAMICS

- Clearance of milrinone varies with individual infants as well as across several gestation.
- It is primarily eliminated via renal route. Hence, there is a chance of delayed renal clearance in renal failure cases, especially when PPHN is associated with perinatal asphyxia.

■ ROUTE

Intravenous

■ DOSE AND MAXIMUM DOSE

Initial dose 0.2–0.33 µg/kg/min; maximum dose 1 µg/kg/min; due to fear of systemic hypotension loading dose should be avoided.

■ ADVERSE EFFECT, CAUTION, PRECAUTIONS AND RED FLAGS

- Systemic hypotension, therefore, 5%–10% adequate vascular volume should be achieved prior to milrinone therapy.
- Arrhythmias are reported occasionally.
- Blood pressure, heart rate, and rhythm should be monitored during infusion of milrinone.
- Caution should be executed in renal failure.
- Thrombocytopenia can happen in 5%–10% cases.

■ TEMPLATE PRESCRIPTION WITH AN EXAMPLE

Diluted with compatible solution (5%–10% dextrose or normal saline with maximum concentration being 200 µg/mL. An example is provided as below:

Drug	Quantity	Diluted in	Total volume	Infusion rate/dose
Inj. Milrinone (1 mL = 1 mg)	Take (3 × weight) mg	5% dextrose/10% dextrose/normal saline	50 mL	1 mL/h = 1 µg/kg/min

■ FURTHER READING

1. Chang AC, Atz AM, Wernovsky G, Burke RP, Wessel DL. Milrinone: systemic and pulmonary hemodynamic effects in neonates after cardiac surgery. 1995;23(11):1907-14.
2. McNamara PJ, Shivananda SP, Sahni M, Freeman D, Taddio A. Pharmacology of milrinone in neonates with persistent pulmonary hypertension of the newborn and suboptimal response to inhaled nitric oxide. Pediatr Crit Care Med. 2013;14(1):74-84.

Bosentan

■ TRADE NAMES, FORMULATION

Available in oral form in strength of 62.5 mg tab from the following brands in Indian market: Bosentan-62.5, Bosentas, Bosentime

■ INDICATIONS

Its use as an adjuvant in acute PPHN (persistent pulmonary hypertension) refractory to inhaled nitric oxide (iNO) and other therapeutic agents in neonates is still evolving. However, it is occasionally used as primary therapy/add-on therapy in chronic pulmonary hypertension secondary to congenital diaphragmatic hernia (CDH) and bronchopulmonary dysplasia (BPD).

■ PHARMACOKINETICS AND PHARMACODYNAMICS

- It undergoes a first pass mechanism in the liver with a half-life of excretion varying between 4 and 5 hours.
- Simultaneous use of bosentan along with sildenafil elevates the former drug while decreasing concentration of the later.

■ ROUTE

Oral

■ DOSE AND MAXIMUM DOSE

1–2 mg/kg twice daily per orally

■ CAUTION, PRECAUTIONS, AND RED FLAGS

Due to risk of hepatotoxicity in prolonged use need to be monitored liver function tests (LFTs) regularly before as well as during therapy.

■ CONTRAINDICATIONS

Preexisting hepatic failure and transaminitis

■ ADVERSE EFFECTS

Hepatotoxicity, anemia

■ TEMPLATE PRESCRIPTION WITH AN EXAMPLE

Currently, it is available in tablet form only in India since its use in children and neonates is still evolving. Tablets need to be made sachets from pharmacy or diluted in 10 mL saline to make a concentration of 6.25 mg/mL which needs to be administered @ 0.5 mL BD to a 3 kg neonate to achieve a dose of 1 mg/kg/dose twice a day.

■ FURTHER READING

1. Abman SH, Hansmann G, Archer SL, Ivy DD, Adatia I, Chung WK, et al. Pediatric Pulmonary Hypertension. Circulation. 2015;132(21):2037-99.

Steroids

Dexamethasone

■ TRADE NAMES

Baycadron, Biodexon, Decadron, Dexamethasone Intensol, Dexasone, Dexalab, Dexona, Soldex, and Solurex

■ INDICATIONS

- Prevention of bronchopulmonary dysplasia in preterm neonates
- Treatment of postintubation laryngeal edema and aid in extubation.

■ RELEVANT PHARMACODYNAMICS AND PHARMACOKINETICS OF THE DRUG

- Long-acting glucocorticoid with biological half-life being 36–54 hours
- No mineralocorticoid activity
- Dexamethasone is approximately 77% protein-bound in plasma. Most of the protein-binding is with serum albumin.
- Dexamethasone is <10% eliminated in urine.

■ AVAILABLE FORMULATIONS

Injection 4 mg/mL (5 mL vial)

■ ROUTE

Intravenous

■ DOSE AND DURATION (INCLUDE THE MAXIMUM DOSE FOR NEONATES)

Postnatal course to the neonate:
- *Prevention of chronic lung disease:* A moderately early-initiated (8–14 days), medium cumulative dose (2–4 mg/kg), short course of systemic dexamethasone is preferred.
  - *Low-dose (DART) protocol:*
    - 0.075 mg/kg/dose 12 hourly for 3 days

- ♦ 0.05 mg/kg/dose 12 hourly for 3 days
- ♦ 0.025 mg/kg/dose 12 hourly for 2 days
- ♦ 0.01 mg/kg/dose 12 hourly for 2 days then stop
  - *High-dose protocol:*
    - ♦ 0.25 mg/kg/dose 12 hourly for 3 days
    - ♦ 0.15 mg/kg/dose 12 hourly for 3 days
    - ♦ 0.1 mg/kg/dose 12 hourly for 3 days
    - ♦ 0.05 mg/kg/dose 12 hourly for 3 days
    - ♦ 0.025 mg/kg/dose 12 hourly for 6 days then stop
  - *Total cumulative dose:*
    - ♦ Low-dose (DART) protocol: 0.89 mg/kg
    - ♦ High-dose protocol: 3.6 mg/kg
- *Extubation/airway edema:*
  - 0.25 mg/kg 8 hourly for up to 3 doses
  - First dose to be given at least 4 hours before extubation
  - *Total cumulative dose:*
    - ♦ Extubation protocol: 0.75 mg/kg
  - Maximum daily dose of dexamethasone: 0.75 mg/kg

ADMINISTRATION

Intravenous: Administered over 3–5 minutes.

PREPARATION

Intravenous: Take 0.5 mL (2 mg) and add 9.5 mL sodium chloride 0.9% to make a final volume of 10 mL with a concentration of 0.2 mg/mL. If volume is too small, further dilute: draw up 1 mL of solution (0.2 mg of dexamethasone) and add 9 mL of sodium chloride 0.9% to make a final volume of 10 mL with a concentration of 0.02 mg/mL.

SOLUTION COMPATIBILITY AND INTERACTIONS

Dexamethasone is compatible with sodium chloride as well as glucose solutions (D5W and D10W).

Y-site: Incompatible with calcium chloride, calcium gluconate, caspofungin, chlorpromazine, ciprofloxacin, dobutamine, erythromycin, esmolol, gentamicin, glycopyrrolate, haloperidol lactate, labetalol, levomepromazine, magnesium sulfate, midazolam, mycophenolate mofetil, pentamidine, phentolamine, promethazine, protamine, rocuronium, tobramycin.

CONTRAINDICATIONS

Untreated systemic infections

■ PRECAUTIONS

- Early (<8 days) treatment, higher dose and longer courses should be avoided to reduce adverse effects.
- Concurrent use with NSAIDs (nonsteroidal anti-inflammatory drugs) for patent ductus arteriosus (PDA) treatment to be avoided.

■ ADVERSE EFFECTS

- *Short-term adverse effects:* Gastrointestinal bleeding, intestinal perforation, hyperglycemia, hypertension, hypertrophic cardiomyopathy, severe retinopathy of prematurity, and growth failure
- *Other effects:*
  - Hypertriglyceridemia
  - Increase in total and immature neutrophil counts
  - Increase in platelet count
  - Adrenal insufficiency, myocardial hypertrophy, and outflow obstruction with higher doses and prolonged courses of dexamethasone
  - Increased risk of infection

■ MONITORING

- Blood glucose levels at least daily
- Blood pressure at least daily

■ TEMPLATE PRESCRIPTION WITH AN EXAMPLE

Dexamethasone (1 mL = 4 mg)

If DART treatment is planned for 1.2 kg neonate, 0.075 mg/kg/dose 12 hourly IV is given for 3 days = 0.09 mg/dose.

Dilution: 0.5 mL (2 mg) dexamethasone and 9.5 mL sodium chloride 0.9% are mixed to make a final volume of 10 mL with a concentration of 0.2 mg/mL.

1 mL of this solution (0.2 mg of dexamethasone) and 9 mL of sodium chloride 0.9% are mixed to make a final volume of 10 mL with a concentration of 0.02 mg/mL.

Required dose: 4.5 mL of this solution (0.02 mg/mL) is given over 15 minutes to give the required 0.09 mg dose.

■ FURTHER READING

1. Harriet Lane Service (Johns Hopkins Hospital); Hughes HK, Kahl LK. Harriet Lane Handbook: A Manual for Pediatric House Officers, 21st edition. St. Louis: Elsevier Health Sciences; 2018.
2. Ramaswamy VV, Bandyopadhyay T, Nanda D, Bandiya P, Ahmed J, Garg A, et al. Assessment of Postnatal Corticosteroids for the Prevention of Bronchopulmonary Dysplasia in Preterm Neonates: A Systematic Review and Network Meta-analysis. JAMA Pediatr. 2021;175:e206826.

Hydrocortisone

■ TRADE NAMES

- *Intravenous:* Solu-Cortef, Cortef, Recorte, Supracort, Drosone, Eflomax, and Hydrowin.
- *Oral:* Hysone.

■ INDICATIONS

- Treatment of vasopressor resistant hypotension
- Treatment of adrenal insufficiency/congenital adrenal hyperplasia
- Treatment of persistent hypoglycemia due to cortisol deficiency

■ RELEVANT PHARMACODYNAMICS AND PHARMACOKINETICS OF THE DRUG

- Hydrocortisone is a corticosteroid, agonist at both glucocorticoid and mineralocorticoid receptors with a biological half-life of <3 hours in term and preterm neonates (for a glucocorticoid activity of 20 mg, equivalent mineralocorticoid activity is 1 mg).
- Hydrocortisone has low-potency relative to synthetic corticosteroids.
- Onset of action of IV preparation is 1–2 hours and absorption is rapid.
- Oral bioavailability is good (>95%); transporter protein P-glycoprotein (P-gp)/ABCB1 influences distribution and bioavailability.
- More than 90% is protein-bound.
- Metabolized in liver via CYP3A4 and excreted in urine.

■ AVAILABLE FORMULATIONS

- *Injection:* 100 mg vial
- *Oral:* 4 mg, 20 mg tablets

■ ROUTE

- Intravenous
- Oral

DOSE (ORAL/INTRAVENOUS) AND DURATION

		Body surface area (BSA) based dosing	Body weight-based dosing	Duration
Vasopressor-resistant hypotension		25–30 mg/m^2/day	• ≥35 weeks postmenstrual age (PMA): 1 mg/kg/dose 6–8 hourly • <35 weeks PMA: 1 mg/kg/dose 6–12 hourly	Guided by cardiovascular response; stopped once perfusion improves
Adrenal insufficiency	• Stress dose	• 100 mg/m^2 bolus followed by 50–100 mg/m^2/day in four divided doses (6 hourly) • 50–100 mg/m^2		• During shock/illness and stopped once general condition improves.
	• Surgery • Maintenance	• 20 mg/m^2/day		• Before the procedure • Lifelong
Hypoglycemia due to cortisol deficiency			1–2.5 mg/kg/dose every 6 hours	If ACTH stimulation is normal, stop when normoglycemia has been achieved. If suggestive of cortisol deficiency, lifelong supplementation is needed

- *Mosteller formula for body surface area (BSA):*
  Square root of the height (cm) multiplied by the weight (kg) divided by 3,600.

$$\sqrt{\frac{\text{Weight (kg)} \times \text{length (cm)}}{3,600}}$$

- *Approximate BSA according to weight of the neonate:*

Weight	0.6	1	1.4	2	3	4
Body surface area (m^2)	0.08	0.1	0.12	0.15	0.2	0.25

Maximum daily dose of hydrocortisone: 100 mg/m^2/day

■ ADMINISTRATION

- *Intravenous:* Slow IV injection over at least 1 minute; IV is continued till oral intake is possible.
- *Oral:* With feeds

■ PREPARATION

Intravenous: Add 2 mL of water for injection to the 100 mg vial (50 mg/mL). Draw up 1 mL (50 mg) of reconstituted solution and add 4 mL sodium chloride 0.9% to make a final volume of 5 mL with a concentration of 10 mg/mL.

Oral: A 4 mg tablet is cut in halves or quarters (depending on the dose required). The portion of tablet required for the dose is crushed and dispersed in 1–2 mL of sterile water or milk for administration.

■ SOLUTION COMPATIBILITY AND INTERACTIONS

Hydrocortisone is compatible with sodium chloride as well as glucose solutions (D5W and D10W).

Y-site: Incompatible with adrenaline hydrochloride, azathioprine, calcium chloride, ciprofloxacin, colistin, dobutamine, dolasetron, ephedrine, ganciclovir, haloperidol lactate, labetalol, midazolam, mycophenolate mofetil, pentamidine, phenobarbitone, promethazine, protamine, and rocuronium.

■ CONTRAINDICATIONS

Untreated systemic infections and patients with known hypersensitivity to the product and its constituents

■ PRECAUTIONS

- Risk of intestinal perforation when used in preterm infants in the first week, particularly when concurrently used with indomethacin

- Untreated systemic bacterial infections
- Neonates with renal impairment, hypothyroidism, or cardiac disease
- Drug needs to be given in tapering doses after prolonged use (>14 days) due to the possibility of prolonged adrenal suppression.
- There is lack of evidence and hydrocortisone should be avoided or used with caution for treatment of hyperinsulinemic hypoglycemia as there is high risk of adrenal suppression and side effects.

ADVERSE EFFECTS

- Hyperglycemia
- Hypertension
- Gastric irritation, gastrointestinal ulceration, and bleeding
- Intestinal perforation in preterm neonates
- Salt and water retention
- Hypokalemia
- Increased risk of infection due to immunosuppression
- Neutrophilia, thrombocytopenia
- Acute withdrawal after use >14 days can lead to acute adrenal insufficiency
- *Long-term:* Disrupted somatic growth, osteopenia

MONITORING

- Blood pressure and blood glucose at least once during illness
- In babies with adrenal insufficiency and treated with hydrocortisone, growth velocity, body weight, and blood pressure to be monitored.

TEMPLATE PRESCRIPTION WITH AN EXAMPLE

Hydrocortisone (1 mL = 100 mg)

If stress dose is planned for 2 kg neonate with adrenal insufficiency and length of 50 cm, 50 mg/m^2 is to be given IV.

BSA according to Mosteller formula is:

$$\sqrt{\frac{2\,(kg) \times 50\,(cm)}{3,600}} = 0.16\,m^2$$

Dose to be given is 50 × 0.16 = 8 mg

Dilution: Add 2 mL of water for injection to the 100-mg vial (50 mg/mL); draw up 1 mL (50 mg) of reconstituted solution and add 4 mL of sodium chloride 0.9% to make a final volume of 5 mL with a concentration of 10 mg/mL.

Required dose: 0.8 mL of this solution (1 mg/mL) is given slow IV over 1 minute.

■ FURTHER READING

1. Harriet Lane Service (Johns Hopkins Hospital); Hughes HK, Kahl LK. Harriet Lane Handbook: A Manual for Pediatric House Officers, 21st edition. St. Louis: Elsevier Health Sciences; 2018.
2. Whittle E, Falhammar H. Glucocorticoid Regimens in the Treatment of Congenital Adrenal Hyperplasia: A Systematic Review and Meta-Analysis. J Endocr Soc 2019;3:1227-45.

Fludrocortisone

■ TRADE NAMES

Oral: Floricot, Florinef tablets

■ INDICATIONS

- Adrenal insufficiency requiring mineralocorticoid replacement
- Salt-losing forms of congenital adrenal hyperplasia

■ RELEVANT PHARMACODYNAMICS AND PHARMACOKINETICS OF THE DRUG

- Fludrocortisone is a synthetic mineralocorticoid used to replace endogenous aldosterone.
- It acts on the kidneys and increases both sodium reabsorption and potassium excretion.
- Its effects are exerted at the transcriptional level.
- A single dose of fludrocortisone may work over the course of 1–2 days despite a relatively short plasma half-life.
- Absorption of fludrocortisone following oral administration is rapid and complete.
- Fludrocortisone is 70–80% protein-bound in plasma, mostly to albumin- and corticosteroid-binding globulin.
- Fludrocortisone is metabolized in the liver by the CYP3A family and is not recommended to be given with strong inhibitors/inducers of CYP3A.

■ AVAILABLE FORMULATIONS

Oral: Fludrocortisone acetate 100 μg tablets

■ ROUTE

Oral

■ DOSE (ORAL) AND DURATION

50–200 μg once a day given lifelong for mineralocorticoid replacement

Maximum daily dose of fludrocortisone: 400 μg/day

■ ADMINISTRATION

Oral: With feeds or immediately after feeds

■ PREPARATION

Oral: Fludrocortisone tablet (100 µg) is dispersed in 2 mL of water (100 µg/2 mL = 50 µg/mL).

■ SOLUTION COMPATIBILITY AND INTERACTIONS

Not to be mixed with any other medicines

■ CONTRAINDICATIONS

Hypersensitivity to fludrocortisone

■ PRECAUTIONS

Untreated systemic infections, hypertension, heart failure, and renal impairment

■ ADVERSE EFFECTS

Hypertension, electrolyte imbalance, and severe edema

■ MONITORING

Weight, blood pressure, and serum electrolytes

■ TEMPLATE PRESCRIPTION WITH AN EXAMPLE

- Fludrocortisone (1 tablet = 100 µg)
- *Required dose:* 1 tablet is dispersed in 2 mL of this water and given orally along with feeds.

■ FURTHER READING

1. Dabas A, Vats P, Sharma R, Singh P, Seth A, Jain V, et al. Management of infants with congenital adrenal hyperplasia. Indian Pediatr. 2020;57:159-64.
2. Harriet Lane Service (Johns Hopkins Hospital); Hughes HK, Kahl LK. Harriet Lane Handbook: A Manual for Pediatric House Officers, 21st edition. St. Louis: Elsevier Health Sciences; 2018.

Budesonide

■ TRADE NAMES

Budevin, Budanec, Buderap, Budemec

■ INDICATIONS

Severe bronchopulmonary dysplasia/chronic lung disease

RELEVANT PHARMACODYNAMICS AND PHARMACOKINETICS OF THE DRUG

- Inhaled steroid with strong glucocorticoid and negligible mineralocorticoid activity
- First-pass metabolism in the liver by CYP3A4 enzymes after systemic absorption
- The percentage of the inhaled dose reaching the lung will depend upon the method and delivery of the nebulized budesonide.
- The duration of effect is >12 hours.

■ AVAILABLE FORMULATIONS

0.5 mg/2 mL respules for nebulization.

■ ROUTE

- Early (<8 days) or late (≥8 days) initiated inhaled budesonide (nebulization)
- Intratracheal budesonide with surfactant as vehicle
- Intratracheal budesonide was found to be associated with more successful extubation from invasive ventilation

■ DOSE AND DURATION

- *Inhaled budesonide:* 200–500 µg twice daily for 10–14 days followed by 200 µg once daily till baby is weaned off from oxygen
- *Intratracheal instillation of budesonide:* 250 µg/kg along with 100 mg/kg (no strong evidence) surfactant repeated 8th hourly or as needed till fraction of inspired oxygen (FiO_2) requirement is <40%.

Maximum daily dose: 1,000 µg/day

■ ADMINISTRATION

Inhaled budesonide using in-line (with the respiratory circuit) jet nebulizer or using a spacer device and connected to an air compressor with an adequate air flow.

■ PREPARATION

Remove one respule from the foil pouch. Pour all of the liquid into the nebulizer reservoir. Do not mix other medications with budesonide in the reservoir.

■ SOLUTION COMPATIBILITY AND INTERACTIONS

Not to be mixed with other nebulizable medications

■ PRECAUTIONS

- Known sensitivity to budesonide
- Caution in neonates with fungal and viral infections in the airways

■ ADVERSE EFFECTS

- Candida infection in the oropharynx
- Gastrointestinal (feed intolerance)
- Suppression of the pituitary–adrenal axis

■ MONITORING

Oxygen saturation

■ TEMPLATE PRESCRIPTION WITH AN EXAMPLE

- *Budesonide:* 0.5 mg/2 mL respules
- *Required dose:* 250 µg
  1 mL is poured from the respule to the nebulizer reservoir

■ FURTHER READING

1. Harriet Lane Service (Johns Hopkins Hospital); Hughes HK, Kahl LK. Harriet Lane Handbook: A Manual for Pediatric House Officers, 21st edition. St. Louis: Elsevier Health Sciences; 2018.
2. Ramaswamy VV, Bandyopadhyay T, Nanda D, Bandiya P, Ahmed J, Garg A, et al. Assessment of Postnatal Corticosteroids for the Prevention of Bronchopulmonary Dysplasia in Preterm Neonates: A Systematic Review and Network Meta-analysis. JAMA Pediatr. 2021;175:e206826.

Medications for Sedation and Analgesia

Midazolam

■ TRADE NAMES

Versed, Midzol, Midacip, Midaz, Benzosed

■ INDICATIONS

- Sedation with mechanical ventilation
- Status epilepticus

■ PHARMACOKINETICS AND PHARMACODYNAMICS

- Relatively short-acting benzodiazepine with rapid onset of action.
- Sedative and anticonvulsant properties related to GABA (gamma-aminobutyric acid) accumulation and occupation of benzodiazepine receptor antianxiety properties related to increasing the glycine inhibitory neurotransmitter.
- *Metabolized* by hepatic CYP3A4 to a less active hydroxylated metabolite.
- Drug accumulation may occur with repeated doses, prolonged infusion therapy, or concurrent administration of cimetidine, erythromycin or fluconazole.
- Highly protein-bound.
- Duration of action is 2–6 hours
- *Elimination half-life* is approximately 4–6 hours in term neonates, and quite variable, up to 22 hours, in premature babies and those with impaired hepatic function.
- *Bioavailability* is approximately 36% with oral administration and 50% with sublingual and intranasal administration.
- Midazolam is water-soluble in acidic solutions and becomes lipid-soluble at physiologic pH.

■ AVAILABLE FORMULATIONS

Injectable

Available: Preservative-free 1- and 5-mg/mL concentrations in 1-, 2-, and 5-mL vials

Also available in an injectable form as 1- and 5-mg/mL concentrations in 1-, 2-, 5-, and 10-mL vials which contain 1% (10 mg/mL) benzyl alcohol as a preservative.

Stability: Stable for 24 hours when diluted with normal saline (NS) or D5W to a concentration of 0.5 mg/mL

Oral

Available: Oral syrup 2 mg/mL

Intranasal availability: Single-dose nasal spray unit delivers 5 mg of midazolam in 0.1 mL of solution

Other routes: Injectable formulation was used for intranasal, buccal, or rectal administration

■ DOSE AND MAXIMUM DOSE

Sedation
Intravenous (IV): 0.05–0.15 mg/kg; repeat as required, usually every 2–4 hours; may also be given intramuscular (IM); dosage requirements are decreased by concurrent use of narcotics.

Continuous IV infusion: 0.1–0.2 mg/kg over 2–5 minutes, followed by 0.03–0.4 mg/kg/h; some recommend 0.03 mg/kg/h for those <32 weeks gestational age and 0.06 mg/kg/h for those older than 32 weeks.

Adjust dosage in patients with hepatic dysfunction; patients with chronic renal failure and/or congestive heart failure eliminate midazolam more slowly, but no dosage adjustment is required in renal dysfunction.

Anticonvulsant

Loading dose: 0.15 mg/kg (150 µg/kg) IV, followed by maintenance dose.

Maintenance infusion: 0.06–0.4 mg/kg/h (1–7 µg/kg/min)

Intranasal: 0.2–0.3 mg/kg per dose using 5-mg/mL injectable form.

Sublingual: 0.2 mg/kg per dose using 5-mg/mL injectable form mixed with a small amount of flavored syrup.

Oral: 0.25 mg/kg per dose

■ CONTRAINDICATIONS

Hypersensitivity to midazolam

■ PRECAUTIONS

Cardiovascular: Hypotension is common when used in conjunction with narcotics, or following rapid bolus administration. Serious cardiorespiratory events, including cardiac arrest resulting in death or permanent injury, have been reported with use of midazolam.

Endocrine or metabolic: Use particular caution in uncompensated acute illness (e.g., severe fluid or electrolyte disturbances).

Respiratory: Serious respiratory events including respiratory depression, airway obstruction, oxygen desaturation, apnea, respiratory arrest, sometimes resulting in death or permanent injury have been reported with use of midazolam; the risk is greatest in those with chronic obstructive pulmonary disease, chronic disease states, or decreased pulmonary reserve, and concomitant use of barbiturates, alcohol, or other central nervous system (CNS) depressants.

Neurologic: CNS depression may occur; increased risk with concomitant use of CNS depressants (opioids), barbiturates, and moderate or strong CYP3A4 inhibitors.

Brain development in children may be affected by repeated or lengthy use of general anesthetic and sedation drugs during surgeries or procedures, especially in children.

Special populations: Gasping syndrome or other severe or fatal adverse effects can occur in neonates and low-birth-weight infants, as formulation contains benzyl alcohol.

■ ADMINISTRATION AND EXAMPLE OF PRESCRIPTION

Intravenous: Administer slow IV push over 10 minutes at a concentration of 1–5 mg/mL. The recommended standard neonatal concentration is 1 mg/mL. For continuous IV infusion may dilute in normal saline (NS) or D5W to a concentration of 0.5 mg/mL. Caution should be taken to avoid intra-arterial injection or extravasation.

Calculation:

Drug	Dose	Dilute in	1 mL/h will give	Range
Midazolam	3 mg/kg	50 mL D5/NS	1 µg/kg/min	1–5 µg/kg/min

Fentanyl

■ TRADE NAMES

Fendrop, Fenilate, Fenstud, Fent, Trofentyl, Verfen, Themifent

■ INDICATIONS

Analgesia, anesthesia, or sedation

■ PHARMACOKINETICS AND PHARMACODYNAMICS

- Synthetic opioid narcotic
- 50–100 times more potent than morphine on a weight basis
- Highly protein-bound (80–85%)
- Extremely lipid-soluble
- Penetrates the central nervous system (CNS) rapidly
- Metabolized extensively in the liver by CYP3A4 enzyme system
- Excreted by the kidney
- Distribution half-life of 3–5 minutes
- Higher clearance and longer half-life in infants compared with children and adults.
- *Half-life:* 8.4 hours when administered as 1 µg/kg/h continuous infusion and 26.7 hours when administered 1 µg/kg/dose intravenous (IV) every 4 hours.

■ AVAILABLE FORMULATIONS

- *Injection:* 50 µg/mL available as 2 mL and 10 mL ampoule
- *Transdermal patch:* 12.5, 25, 50, 75, 100 µg/h

■ ROUTE

Intravenouse (IV).

■ DOSE AND MAXIMUM DOSE

- *Analgesia:*
  - *Single or intermittent dose:* 0.5–3 µg/kg/dose slow IV push; repeat as required (usually every 2–4 hours)
  - *Continuous infusion:* 0.5–2 µg/kg/h; tolerance may develop rapidly following constant infusion
- *Anesthesia:* 5–50 µg/kg per dose.
- *Sedation:*
  - *Single or intermittent dose:* 0.5–4 µg/kg per dose; repeat as required (usually every 2–4 hours)

- *Continuous infusion:* 1–5 µg/kg/h; tolerance may develop rapidly following constant infusion.
- *Maximum dose:* 100 µg/dose

◼ CAUTION, PRECAUTIONS, AND RED FLAGS

- *Life-threatening respiratory depression/apnea:* Especially during initiation of fentanyl or following a dose increase; an opioid antagonist, intubation equipment, and oxygen should be available.
- *Cytochrome P450 3A4 interaction:* The concomitant use of fentanyl with all cytochrome P450 3A4 inhibitors may result in an increase in fentanyl plasma concentrations, which could increase or prolong adverse drug effects and may cause potentially fatal respiratory depression.
- Concomitant use of opioids with benzodiazepines or other CNS depressants may result in profound sedation, respiratory depression, coma, and death.
- *Look-alike, sound-alike drug names:* FentaNYL citrate was confused with SUFentanil citrate.

◼ ADMINISTRATION AND EXAMPLE OF PRESCRIPTION

- *Solution compatibility:* D5W and NS
- 1 mL of commercially available injection fentanyl contains 50 µg of fentanyl. In a baby weighing 2.5 kg, if we want to start fentanyl at a rate of 2 µg/kg/h = 2 × 2.5 = 5 µg/h = 5 × 24 = 120 µg/day = 2.4 mL/day
- It means if we add 2.4 mL of fentanyl in 24 mL of fluid and give @ rate of 1 mL/h with syringe pump, we will give fentanyl at @ 2 µg/kg/h.
  Some easier to use formulae are mentioned in the following text.

Formula 1:
- Take 2.5 mL/kg of fentanyl and add D5 to it to make the final volume 25 mL. 1 mL/h of this solution is equivalent to 5 µg/kg/h.
- Example for a 2.5 kg baby 2.5 mL/kg = 2.5 × 2.5 = 6.25 mL fentanyl to be added to D5 to make final volume 25 mL. 1 mL/h of this solution is equivalent to 5 µg/kg/h.

Formula 2:
- Take 50 mg/kg of fentanyl in 24 mL D5. 1 mL/h of this solution is equivalent to 2 µg/kg/h.
- Example for 2.5 kg baby 50 mg/kg = 50 × 2.5 = 125 mg fentanyl to be added D5 to make final volume 25 mL. 1 mL/h of this solution is equivalent to 2 µg/kg/h.

Formula 3:

- $$50 \times \frac{\text{Desired dose } (\mu g/kg/h)}{\text{Desired infusion rate } (mL/h)} \times \text{Wt (kg)} \frac{\mu g \text{ Fentanyl}}{50 \text{ mL fluid}}$$

- Example for a 2.5 kg baby if desired dose is 2 µg/kg/h and infusion rate desired is 1 mL/h.

- $$\frac{50 \times 2 \times 2.5}{1} = 250 \text{ µg fentanyl in 50 mL fluid}$$

CONTRAINDICATIONS

Because of the risk of respiratory depression, fentanyl is contraindicated for use as an as-needed analgesic, in nonopioid tolerant patients, in acute pain, and in postoperative pain.

ADVERSE EFFECTS

- Respiratory depression occurs when anesthetic doses (>5 µg/kg) are used.
- Chest wall rigidity has occurred in 4% of neonates who received 2.2–6.5 µg/kg per dose, occasionally associated with laryngospasm. Rigidity may be prevented by concomitant use of neuromuscular blocking agents with mechanical ventilation.
- Naloxone reverses respiratory depression and chest wall rigidity.
- Urinary retention may occur when using continuous infusions.
- Significant withdrawal symptoms have been reported in patients treated with continuous infusion for 5 days or longer.
- Tolerance may develop to analgesic doses with prolonged use.

MONITORING AND PRECAUTIONS

- Monitor respiratory and cardiovascular status closely
- Monitor for respiratory depression, especially during initiation of fentanyl or following a dose increase.
- Observe for abdominal distention, loss of bowel sounds, and muscle rigidity.
- The concomitant use of fentanyl with all cytochrome P450 3A4 inhibitors may result in an increase in fentanyl plasma concentrations.

FURTHER READING

1. Harriet Lane Service (Johns Hopkins Hospital); Kleinman K, McDaniel L, Molloy M. The Harriet Lane Handbook: A Manual for Pediatric House Officers, 22nd edition. Philadelphia: Elsevier; 2021.
2. IBM Micromedex NeoFax and Pediatric Drug Available from: https://www.merative.com/micromedex-training-center/neofax-peds [Last accessed March, 2024].
3. Phelps SJ, Hagemann TM, Lee KR, Thompson AJ. Pediatric Injectable Drugs (The Teddy Bear Book), 11th edition. United States: American Society of Health-System Pharmacists; 2018.

Morphine

■ TRADE NAMES

Morphine, Relimorf, Verve, Morphitroy, San-Morf, Vermor

■ INDICATIONS

- Analgesia/procedural pain
- Neonatal abstinence syndrome
- Opioid dependence

■ PHARMACOKINETICS AND PHARMACODYNAMICS

- Narcotic analgesic that stimulates brain opioid receptors
- Increases venous capacitance, caused by release of histamine and central suppression of adrenergic tone
- Gastrointestinal (GI) secretions and motility decreased; increases smooth muscle tone
- *Half-life:* Approximately 9 hours for morphine and 18 hours for morphine-6-glucuronide; steady state concentrations of morphine are reached by 24–48 hours.

■ AVAILABLE FORMULATIONS

- *Injection:* 10 mg/mL and 15 mg/mL ampoule
- Tablet/capsule/syrup/gel

■ ROUTE

- Intravenous (IV)
- Oral

■ DOSE AND MAXIMUM DOSE

- *Analgesia:*
  - *Continuous infusion:* Loading dose 100 µg/kg IV followed by 10 µg/kg/h; postoperatively may be increased further to 20 µg/kg/h
  - There is insufficient evidence to support the routine use of opioids in mechanically ventilated neonates to reduce pain in a systematic review.
- *Neonatal abstinence syndrome:*
  - Initial dose: 0.03–0.1 mg/kg per dose orally every 3–4 hours; maximum dose 0.2 mg/kg; wean dose by 10–20% every 2–3 days based on abstinence scoring

- Sublingual buprenorphine was associated with the largest reduction in length of treatment and length of stay for neonatal abstinence syndrome (NAS) compared to clonidine, diluted tincture of opium and clonidine, diluted tincture of opium, morphine, methadone, and phenobarbital.
- Methadone outperformed morphine for the treatment of NAS.

■ CAUTION, PRECAUTIONS, AND RED FLAGS

- Monitor respiratory and cardiovascular status closely.
- Observe for abdominal distention and loss of bowel sounds; consider urine retention if output is decreased.
- Renal clearance markedly decreased in hypoxic ischemic encephalopathy (HIE) babies receiving hypothermia.
- *Terminal injection site incompatibility:* Azithromycin, cefepime, pentobarbital, and phenytoin
- Rapid intravenous administration may result in chest wall rigidity.
- Use caution in patients susceptible to intracranial effects of carbon dioxide retention.

■ ADMINISTRATION AND EXAMPLE OF PRESCRIPTION

- *Solution compatibility:* D5W, D10W, and normal saline (NS)
- 1 mL of commercially available injection morphine contains 10 mg of morphine; in a baby weighing 2.5 kg if we want to start morphine at a rate of 20 µg/kg/h = 20 × 2.5 µg/h = 50 µg/h = 50 × 24 = 1,200 µg/day = 0.12 mL/day
- If we add 0.12 mL of morphine in 24 mL of fluid and give @ rate of 1 mL/h with syringe pump, we will give morphine at rate of 20 µg/kg/h.

Some easier formula: Take 1 mg/kg of morphine and add to D5 to make final volume 24 mL. 1 mL/h of this solution is equivalent to 40 µg/kg/h.

■ CONTRAINDICATIONS

- Significant respiratory depression
- Known or suspected gastrointestinal obstruction including paralytic ileus

■ ADVERSE EFFECTS

- Rapid intravenous administration may result in chest wall rigidity.
- *Neurologic:* Impaired consciousness or coma, potentially life-threatening serotonin syndrome
- Naloxone should be readily available to reverse adverse effects.

■ MONITORING AND PRECAUTIONS

Preexisting circulatory shock may reduce cardiac output and blood pressure. Severe hypotension, including orthostatic hypotension and syncope, in ambulatory patients may occur; especially in patients with compromised ability to maintain blood pressure; monitoring recommended.

■ FURTHER READING

1. Harriet Lane Service (Johns Hopkins Hospital); Kleinman K, McDaniel L, Molloy M. The Harriet Lane Handbook: A Manual for Pediatric House Officers, 22nd edition. Philadelphia: Elsevier; 2021.
2. IBM Micromedex NeoFax and Pediatric Drug Available from: https://www.merative.com/micromedex-training-center/neofax-peds [Last accessed March, 2024].
3. Phelps SJ, Hagemann TM, Lee KR, Thompson AJ. Pediatric Injectable Drugs (The Teddy Bear Book), 11th edition. United States: American Society of Health-System Pharmacists; 2018.

Antimicrobials

Ampicillin

▌ RELEVANT PHARMACODYNAMICS AND PHARMACOKINETICS

A semisynthetic penicillin which is bactericidal in action; excretion is mainly by renal route. Clearance is related inversely with postnatal age. Half-life in term infants <7 days is 4 hours.

■ DOSE

- 25–50 mg/kg/dose by intravenous (IV) slow push or intramuscular (IM).
- *Postmenstrual age (PMA) ≤29 weeks*: 25–50 mg/kg/dose every 12 hourly in postnatal 0–28 days; 25–50 mg/kg/dose every 8 hourly in postnatal >28 days.
- *PMA 30–36 weeks*: 25–50 mg/kg/dose every 12 hourly in postnatal 0–14 days; 25–50 mg/kg/dose every 8 hourly in postnatal >14 days.
- *PMA 37–44 weeks*: 25–50 mg/kg/dose every 12 hourly in postnatal 0–7 days; 25–50 mg/kg/dose every 8 hourly in postnatal >7 days.
- *PMA ≥45 weeks*: 25–50 mg/kg/dose every 6 hourly.

  In meningitis, the dose in ≤7 postnatal days is 100 mg/kg/dose IV every 8 hours and in >7 postnatal days is 75 mg/kg/dose IV every 6 hours.

■ ADMINISTRATION

Intravenous: Doses 500 mg or less should be administered slowly over 3–5 minutes IV and over at least 10–15 minutes for doses 1 g or greater.

Intramuscular: Mix to a final concentration of 250 mg/mL for IM administration.

■ SOLUTION COMPATIBILITY

D5W, D5W in 0.45% sodium chloride, lactated Ringer's solution, NS, sterile water

■ SOLUTION INCOMPATIBILITY

Amikacin, amiodarone, dopamine, epinephrine, fluconazole, gentamicin, hydralazine, metoclopramide, midazolam, nicardipine, sodium bicarbonate, and tobramycin

■ INDICATIONS

Bacterial meningitis caused by *Listeria*, group B streptococci, and other gram-negative bacteria; septicemia caused by susceptible gram-positive organisms including penicillin G-susceptible staphylococci, and enterococci; gram-negative sepsis caused by *Escherichia coli*, *Proteus mirabilis*, and *Salmonella* and species

■ CONTRAINDICATIONS/PRECAUTIONS

Hypersensitivity to penicillin derivatives

■ ADVERSE EFFECTS

Central nervous system excitation or seizure activity with high doses. Prolongation of bleeding times (by approximately 60 seconds) has been reported after the third or fourth dose in neonates 33–41 weeks gestational age (GA) receiving 50–100 mg/kg every 12 hours; rarely, hypersensitivity reactions (maculopapular rash, urticarial rash, or fever) in neonates

■ MONITORING AND PRECAUTIONS

Monitoring of renal, hepatic, and hematopoietic function in patients receiving prolonged treatment.

■ FURTHER READING

1. NeoFax® Drug Monograph Summary, AIIMS Neonatal Clinical Protocols.

Amoxicillin

RELEVANT PHARMACODYNAMICS AND PHARMACOKINETICS

It is a semisynthetic antibiotic inhibiting the biosynthesis of the cell wall. It has bactericidal action against most strains of gram-positive and gram-negative microorganisms. After administration, time to peak concentration is achieved in 1–2 hours. Distribution is wide in most body tissues and fluids, except brain and spinal fluid, however, brain penetration may occur with inflamed meninges.

DOSE

- Maximum 30 mg/kg/day orally divided every 12 hours
- 100 mg/kg/day orally in two divided doses in neonates 2 kg or more and 75 mg/kg/day orally in two divided doses in neonates <2 kg have been used in infants 0–59 days with possible serious infections.

Urinary tract infection, prophylaxis: 10–15 mg/kg/day orally once daily

ADMINISTRATION

Shake well before measuring the dose; may mix the dose with formula, milk.

INDICATIONS

- Genitourinary infections
- Skin and skin structure infections caused by *Streptococcus* and *Staphylococcus*
- Lower respiratory tract infections caused by *Streptococcus* and *Staphylococcus* hemolytic strains

CONTRAINDICATIONS/PRECAUTIONS

Gastrointestinal: *Clostridium difficile*-associated diarrhea, including mild diarrhea to fatal colitis.

Immunologic: Severe anaphylactic reactions, including fatalities especially in patients with a history of penicillin hypersensitivity.

Mononucleosis: Avoid use due to a high risk of developing an erythematous skin rash.

Renal: Severe renal impairment [glomerular filtration rate (GFR) <30 mL/min] or hemodialysis; dose adjustment recommended

ADVERSE EFFECTS

Rash, diarrhea, and vomiting

FURTHER READING

1. NeoFax® Drug Monograph Summary, AIIMS Neonatal Clinical Protocols.

Amikacin

RELEVANT PHARMACODYNAMICS AND PHARMACOKINETICS

Aminoglycoside binds to 16S rRNA and the RNA-binding S12 protein of the 30S subunit of prokaryotic ribosome. It inhibits protein synthesis. It is given parentally as its oral absorption is poor. Peak serum concentration is reached in half to 2 hours. Half-life is around 2 hours.

DOSE

- *Postmenstrual age (PMA) ≤29 weeks:* The dose is 18 mg/kg every 48 hourly in postnatal 0–7 days; 15 mg/kg every 36 hourly in postnatal 8–28 days; and 15 mg/kg every 24 hourly in postnatal ≥29 days.
- *PMA 30–34:* The dose is 18 mg/kg every 36 hourly in postnatal 0–7 days; 15 mg/kg every 24 hourly in postnatal ≥8 days; and 15 mg/kg every 24 hourly in postnatal day ≥29 days.
- *PMA ≥35:* The dose is 15 mg/kg every 24 hourly.

ADMINISTRATION

- Intravenous (IV) or intramuscular (IM)
- Dilute to a final concentration of 2.5–10 mg/mL and administer as IV infusion by syringe pump over 60–120 minutes.
- Administer as a separate infusion from penicillin-containing compounds. IM injection is associated with variable absorption, especially in preterm neonates.

SOLUTION COMPATIBILITY

Normal saline, 5% dextrose, and 10% dextrose

SOLUTION INCOMPATIBILITY

It is incompatible with lipid emulsion. Amphotericin B, ampicillin, azithromycin, heparin (at concentrations >1 U/mL), imipenem/cilastatin, oxacillin, phenytoin, and ticarcillin/clavulanate.

INDICATIONS

Gram-negative bacilli that are resistant to other aminoglycosides. It is used along with beta-lactam antibiotic for neonatal sepsis and other severe infections because of the possibility of infections due to gram-positive organisms such as streptococci or pneumococci

■ CONTRAINDICATIONS/PRECAUTIONS

Mixing of aminoglycosides with beta-lactam antibiotics (penicillin or cephalosporins) may result in a significant mutual inactivation.

Gastrointestinal: Clostridium difficile-associated diarrhea; immunologic: allergic-type reactions

Monitor clinically for ototoxicity and nephrotoxicity.

■ ADVERSE EFFECTS

These include transient and reversible renal tubular dysfunction, ototoxicity, and increased neuromuscular blockade when used with pancuronium or other neuromuscular blocking agents.

■ FURTHER READING

1. NeoFax® Drug Monograph Summary. AIIMS Neonatal Clinical Protocols.

Gentamicin

▌ RELEVANT PHARMACODYNAMICS AND PHARMACOKINETICS

Volume of distribution is increased, and clearance is decreased in patients with patent ductus arteriosus (PDA). Serum half-life is prolonged in premature and asphyxiated newborns. Inactivation of gentamicin by penicillin-containing compounds appears to be a time-, temperature-, and concentration-dependent process. Dosing is based on the fact that there is postantibiotic effect on bacterial killing, especially when treating concurrently with a beta-lactam antibiotic and there may be less toxicity with less frequent dosing due to less renal drug accumulation.

■ DOSE

- *Postmenstrual age (PMA) ≤29 weeks:* The dose is 5 mg/kg every 48 hourly in postnatal 0–7 days; 4 mg/kg every 36 hourly in postnatal 8–28 days; and 4 mg/kg every 24 hourly in postnatal ≥29 days.
- *PMA 30–34:* The dose is 4.5 mg/kg every 36 hourly in postnatal 0–7 days and 4 mg/kg every 24 hourly in postnatal ≥8 days.
- *PMA ≥35:* The dose is 4 mg/kg every 24 hourly.

■ ADMINISTRATION

Infuse over a period of 30–120 minutes using a concentration of 2 or 10 mg/mL.

Administer as a separate infusion from penicillin-containing compounds. Intramuscular (IM) injection is associated with variable absorption, especially in the very small infant.

■ SOLUTION COMPATIBILITY

D5W, D10W, and NS (normal saline)

■ SOLUTION INCOMPATIBILITY

Amphotericin B, ampicillin, azithromycin, furosemide, imipenem/cilastatin, heparin (concentrations >1 U/mL), indomethacin, mezlocillin, nafcillin, oxacillin, propofol, and ticarcillin/clavulanate.

■ INDICATIONS

Treatment of infections caused by aerobic gram-negative bacilli (e.g., *Klebsiella, Escherichia coli*); usually used in combination with a beta-lactam antibiotic.

■ CONTRAINDICATIONS/PRECAUTIONS

Patients with derange renal function, or those who receive prolonged therapy are at an increased risk of toxicity. Discontinue therapy or adjust dose, if there is evidence of ototoxicity or nephrotoxicity.

■ ADVERSE EFFECTS

Transient and reversible renal tubular dysfunction may occur, resulting in increased urinary losses of sodium, calcium, and magnesium. Vestibular and auditory ototoxicity may occur. Increased neuromuscular blockade (neuromuscular weakness and respiratory failure) may occur when used with pancuronium or other neuromuscular blocking agents.

The use of gentamicin ointment for newborn ocular prophylaxis has been associated with periocular ulcerative dermatitis.

■ MONITORING

Aminoglycoside therapy has been associated with potential neurotoxicity, ototoxicity, and nephrotoxicity.

■ FURTHER READING

1. AIIMS Neonatal protocols
2. Neofax Drug monograph

Cefotaxime

RELEVANT PHARMACODYNAMICS AND PHARMACOKINETICS

Cefotaxime is one of many third-generation cephalosporin antibiotics. The mechanism of action appears to be by bacterial cell wall disruption. Metabolized in the liver to an active compound, desacetylcefotaxime. The drug distributes widely (i.e., cerebrospinal fluid (CSF), bile, bronchial secretions, lung tissue, ascitic fluid, middle ear). Excreted renally as unchanged drug (20%–36%) and active metabolite (15%–25%). Half-life is 3.63 hours (1.67–10.35 hours)

DOSE

The usual dose in sepsis is 50 mg/kg/dose.

- *Postmenstrual age (PMA) <32 weeks:* The dose is 50 mg/kg/dose every 8 hourly in postnatal ≥7 days.
- *PMA ≥32 weeks:* The dose is 50 mg/kg/dose every 6 hourly in postnatal ≥7 days.
- *Any PMA*: The dose is 50 mg/kg/dose every 12 hourly in postnatal <7 days. In meningitis:
  - 0–7 days: 100–150 mg/kg/day intravenous (IV) divided every 8–12 hours; in weight <2 kg consider giving smaller dose and longer interval.
  - More than 8 days: 150–200 mg/kg/day IV divided every 6–8 hours; in weight <2 kg consider giving smaller dose and longer interval.

ADMINISTRATION

It may be given by IM injection, IV push (over 3–5 minutes), or intermittent IV infusion.

For IV push, a concentration of 50–100 mg/mL may be used. For intermittent IV infusion, dilute to a concentration of 10–40 mg/mL and infuse over 10–30 minutes.

SOLUTION COMPATIBILITY

D5W, D10W, and normal saline (NS).

SOLUTION INCOMPATIBILITY

Azithromycin, fluconazole, protamine sulfate, sodium bicarbonate, and vancomycin

■ INDICATIONS

Lower respiratory tract infection (LRTI), gastrointestinal tract (GIT) infections, bacteremia, sepsis, skin, and skin structure infections, intra-abdominal infections, bone and joint infections, and central nervous system (CNS) infection (meningitis, ventriculitis). Suspectable organism-predominantly gram-positive and few gram-negative.

■ CONTRAINDICATIONS/PRECAUTIONS

Extravasation, including extensive perivascular, may occur causing tissue damage requiring surgical intervention. Use cautiously in patients with a history of gastrointestinal disease, especially colitis *Clostridium difficile*-associated diarrhea, ranging from mild diarrhea to fatal colitis, has been reported. Leukopenia, neutropenia, or granulocytopenia and in rare cases bone marrow failure, pancytopenia, or agranulocytosis may occur. Increased risk of allergic reaction including serious reactions requiring medical intervention. Use caution in the presence of renal insufficiency.

■ ADVERSE EFFECTS

Side effects are rare but include rash, phlebitis, diarrhea, leukopenia, granulocytopenia, and eosinophilia.

■ MONITORING

Periodic complete blood count (CBC)

■ FURTHER READING

1. NeoFax® Drug Monograph Summary AIIMS Neonatal Clinical Protocols

Ceftriaxone

■ RELEVANT PHARMACODYNAMICS AND PHARMACOKINETICS

Third-generation cephalosporin with a wider drug distribution in body; half-life varies from 5 to 16 hours in preterm infants. Dose adjustment is required in combined hepatic renal failure.

■ DOSE

- *Sepsis:* 50 mg/kg every 24 hours
- *Meningitis*: 100 mg/kg loading dose, then 80 mg/kg every 24 hours
- *Uncomplicated gonococcal ophthalmia*: 25–50 mg/kg (maximum 125 mg) IV/IM (intravenous/intramuscular) as a single dose

■ ADMINISTRATION

Intravenous: Administer over 60 minutes at a concentration of 10–40 mg/mL (lower concentrations may be used, if necessary). *Do not mix with calcium-containing solutions in the same IV line;* precipitation may occur. If administered within the last 48 hours, avoid calcium-containing products.

■ SOLUTION COMPATIBILITY

Normal saline, 5% dextrose, and 10% dextrose

■ SOLUTION INCOMPATIBILITY

Any calcium-containing solution

■ INDICATIONS

Sepsis, and meningitis caused by susceptible gram-negative organisms (e.g., *Klebsiella, Escherichia coli, Pseudomonas, Haemophilus influenzae*).

■ CONTRAINDICATIONS/PRECAUTIONS

Contraindications: Contraindicated for use in neonates with hyperbilirubinemia; displaces bilirubin from albumin-binding sites, resulting in higher free bilirubin serum concentrations.

Concurrent administration of ceftriaxone and IV calcium-containing solutions (including parenteral nutrition) or products in neonates is contraindicated.

■ ADVERSE EFFECTS

Eosinophilia, thrombocytosis, leukopenia; increase in bleeding time, diarrhea, BUN (blood urea nitrogen), and serum creatinine, AST (aspartate aminotransferase) and ALT (alanine aminotransferase), skin rash; transient gallbladder precipitations occasionally associated with colicky abdominal pain, nausea, and vomiting

■ MONITORING

Frequently monitor coagulation parameters during concomitant vitamin K antagonist therapy, complete blood count (CBC) for eosinophilia, thrombocytosis, leukopenia; serum electrolytes, BUN, creatinine; AST, ALT, bilirubin.

■ FURTHER READING

1. NeoFax® Drug Monograph Summary, AIIMS Neonatal Clinical Protocols.

Ceftazidime

■ RELEVANT PHARMACODYNAMICS AND PHARMACOKINETICS

Ceftazidime is a third-generation cephalosporin with activity against species. It is bactericidal in action and inhibits enzymes responsible for cell wall synthesis. It is widely in body tissues and fluids [i.e., CSF (cerebrospinal fluid), bile, bronchial secretions, lung tissue, ascitic fluid, middle ear]. Protein binding is low (<10%). It is excreted unchanged in the urine (80%–90%). Serum half-life following intravenous (IV) administration is approximately 1.9 hours. Half-life is significantly longer in patients with renal impairment.

■ DOSE

30 mg/kg/dose IV infusion over 30 minutes.

- *Postmenstrual age (PMA) ≤29 weeks:* The dose is 30 mg/kg/dose every 12 hourly in postnatal 0–28 days; 30 mg/kg/dose every 8 hourly in postnatal >28 days
- *PMA 30–36 weeks:* The dose is 30 mg/kg/dose every 12 hourly in postnatal 0–14 days; 30 mg/kg/dose every 8 hourly in postnatal >14 days
- *PMA 37–44 weeks:* The dose is 30 mg/kg/dose every 12 hourly in postnatal 0–7 days; 30 mg/kg/dose every 8 hourly in postnatal >7 days

■ ADMINISTRATION

Intravenous:
- IV push over 3–5 minutes at a maximum concentration of 100 or 200 mg/mL.
- Intermittent IV infusion over 30 minutes at a concentration of 1–40 mg/mL as well as 50 mg/mL.

Intramuscular (IM): Deep IM administration into a large muscle mass for less serious infections

■ SOLUTION COMPATIBILITY

Normal saline, 5% dextrose and 10% dextrose

■ SOLUTION INCOMPATIBILITY

Amiodarone, fluconazole, midazolam, nicardipine, phenytoin, and vancomycin

■ INDICATIONS

Treatment of neonatal meningitis and sepsis caused by susceptible gram-negative organisms (e.g., *Escherichia coli*, *Haemophilus influenzae*, *Neisseria*, *Klebsiella*, and *Proteus* species), especially *Pseudomonas.*

■ CONTRAINDICATIONS/PRECAUTIONS

Dose and duration need to be modified when the renal function is impaired.

■ ADVERSE EFFECTS

Rash, diarrhea, elevated hepatic transaminases, eosinophilia, and positive Coombs' test

■ FURTHER READING

1. NeoFax® Drug Monograph Summary

Cefepime

RELEVANT PHARMACODYNAMICS AND PHARMACOKINETICS

Fourth-generation cephalosporin with treatment efficacy equivalent to third-generation cephalosporins; the drug distributes widely in body tissues and fluids [i.e., CSF (cerebrospinal fluid), bile, bronchial secretions, lung tissue, ascitic fluid, middle ear]. Protein-binding is low (approximately 20%), and it is primarily excreted unchanged in the urine. Serum half-life is approximately 2 hours.

DOSE

- *Term and preterm infants <28 days of age*: 50 mg/kg/dose intravenous (IV) every 12 hours
- *Term and preterm infants 28 days of age and younger*: 30 mg/kg/dose IV every 12 hours
- *Meningitis and severe infections due to Pseudomonas aeruginosa or Enterobacter* sp: 50 mg/kg/dose IV every 12 hours

ADMINISTRATION

- Give as an IV infusion in a compatible solution over 30 minutes
- May be given by IM injection

SOLUTION COMPATIBILITY

D5W, D10W, D5LR, D5NS, and normal saline (NS)

SOLUTION COMPATIBILITY

Acyclovir, aminophylline, amphotericin B, cimetidine, diazepam, dobutamine, dopamine, enalaprilat, famotidine, ganciclovir, magnesium sulfate, metoclopramide, midazolam, morphine, nicardipine, phenytoin, tobramycin, and vancomycin

INDICATIONS

Treatment of serious infections caused by susceptible gram-negative organisms especially *Escherichia coli, Haemophilus influenzae, Neisseria, Klebsiella*, and *Enterobacter* species and *Pseudomonas*. Treatment of serious infections caused by susceptible gram-positive organisms (e.g., *Streptococcus pneumoniae, Streptococcus pyogenes* and *Staphylococcus aureus*)

■ CONTRAINDICATIONS/PRECAUTIONS

Hypersensitivity to cephalosporins or components of the formulation; mainly excreted renally; clearance is reduced in renal failure.

■ ADVERSE EFFECTS

Reported adverse effects are uncommon, but include rash, diarrhea, elevated hepatic transaminases, eosinophilia, and positive Coombs' test.

■ FURTHER READING

1. NeoFax® Drug Monograph Summary, AIIMS Neonatal Clinical Protocols.

Cefoperazone–Sulbactam

▌ RELEVANT PHARMACODYNAMICS AND PHARMACOKINETICS

Third-generation cephalosporin with beta-lactamase inhibitor (sulbactam). The half-life varies between 1.6 and 2.4 hours. Dosage modification is required in the presence of severe biliary obstruction or concomitant renal and hepatic dysfunction, since biliary excretion is the primary route of cefoperazone elimination. It does not penetrate cerebrospinal fluid (CSF).

■ DOSE

30–40 mg/kg/dose of cefoperazone, infusion to be give over 30 minutes to 1 hour every 8 hourly

■ ADMINISTRATION

Give as an intravenous solution with compatible diluent over 30 minutes.

■ SOLUTION COMPATIBILITY

Normal Saline, 5% dextrose and 10% dextrose

■ INDICATIONS

Upper and lower respiratory tract infections, septicemia, skin, and genitourinary infections

■ CONTRAINDICATIONS/PRECAUTIONS

Hypersensitivity; allergy to penicillin

■ ADVERSE EFFECTS

Used with caution in hepatic failure

■ MONITORING AND PRECAUTIONS

Needs to be given with caution in patients with biliary obstruction, receiving anticoagulant therapy, and renal and hepatic impairment.

■ FURTHER READING

1. Harriet Service (Johns Hopkins Hospital); Kleinman K, McDaniel L, Molloy M. The Harriet Lane Handbook: A Manual for Pediatric House Officers, 22nd edition. Philadelphia: Elsevier; 2021.
2. NeoFax® Drug Monograph Summary.

Ciprofloxacin

■ RELEVANT PHARMACODYNAMICS AND PHARMACOKINETICS

Inhibits CYP 450 1A2; ciprofloxacin can increase effects and/or toxicity of caffeine, methotrexate, theophylline, warfarin, tizanidine (excessive sedation and dangerous hypotension), and cyclosporine.

■ DOSE

10 mg/kg/dose Q12th hourly over 30–60 minutes intravenous (IV)

■ ADMINISTRATION

Intravenous, oral

■ SOLUTION COMPATIBILITY

5% dextrose

■ SOLUTION INCOMPATIBILITY

Antacids and divalent salts

■ INDICATIONS

Gram-negative bacterial infection including meningitis; limited use in neonates due to possible adverse effects.

■ CONTRAINDICATIONS/PRECAUTIONS

Use with caution in children aged <18 years (like other quinolones, tendon rupture can occur during or after therapy, especially with concomitant corticosteroid use), alkalinized urine (crystalluria), seizures, excessive sunlight (photosensitivity), and renal dysfunction.

■ ADVERSE EFFECTS

Gastrointestinal upset, renal failure, rash, and seizures; tendon rupture can occur during or after therapy; prolong half-life of aminophylline, theophylline, and caffeine, hence, to be used with caution with these drugs.

■ MONITORING

Complete blood count, renal, and hepatic function during prolonged therapy

■ FURTHER READING

1. AIIMS Neonatal Clinical Protocols.
2. Harriet Service (Johns Hopkins Hospital); Kleinman K, McDaniel L, Molloy M. The Harriet Lane Handbook: A Manual for Pediatric House Officers, 22nd edition. Philadelphia: Elsevier; 2021.

Colistin

■ TRADE NAMES

Colistin/Xylistin/Colistimethate

■ INDICATIONS

Gram-negative infections, multidrug-resistant infections

■ PHARMACOKINETICS AND PHARMACODYNAMICS

- Colistimethate sodium is a surface-active agent that is used to penetrate and disrupt the cell membrane of bacteria.
- Higher serum levels were obtained at 10 minutes following intravenous (IV) administration compared with intramuscular (IM) administration.
- The half-life was 2.6 hours in neonates (0–7 days) and 2.3 hours in infants 7 days or older.

■ AVAILABLE FORMULATIONS

- Each vial containing Colistimethate sodium (pentasodium colistin methanesulfonate) is equivalent to 150 mg of colistin base activity.
- Colistin base 1 mg is equivalent to 2.4 mg of Colistimethate sodium.
- Colistimethate sodium is 12,500 IU/mg and colistin base is 30,000 IU/mg.

■ ROUTE OF ADMINISTRATION

- Intravenous route
- *Intermittent administration:* Infuse one-half of the total daily dose slowly over 3–5 minutes at a concentration of 75 mg/mL colistin base every 12 hours.

■ DOSE AND ADMINISTRATION

- *Gram-negative infections:* 2.5–5 mg/kg/day of colistin base IV or IM in two to four divided doses, depending on severity of infection
- *Maximum:* 5 mg/kg/day of colistin base in patients with normal renal function
- 25,000 IU/kg/dose every 8th hourly

■ SOLUTION COMPATIBILITY

Normal saline (NS), D5NS, D5 0.45% NS, D5W

■ CAUTION, PRECAUTIONS, AND RED FLAGS

Acute respiratory failure may result when reconstituted Colistimethate solution for inhalation is not used promptly.

■ ADVERSE EFFECTS

- *Clostridium difficile*-associated diarrhea (CDAD), including mild diarrhea to fatal colitis, has been reported and may occur >2 months after administration.
- Respiratory arrest has been reported after IM administration.
- Reversible and dose-dependent nephrotoxicity

■ MONITORING

- Close monitoring for urine output blood urea nitrogen (BUN) and serum creatinine is required.
- Monitor vital signs and blood pressure.

■ FURTHER READING

1. Harriet Service (Johns Hopkins Hospital); Kleinman K, McDaniel L, Molloy M. The Harriet Lane Handbook: A Manual for Pediatric House Officers, 22nd edition. Philadelphia: Elsevier; 2021.
2. Young TE, Magnum B. Micromedex NeoFax Essentials. New Jersey: Thomson Reuters; 2020.

Elores

■ INDICATIONS

Elores should be used only to treat or prevent infections that are proven or strongly suspected to be caused by susceptible bacteria, especially multidrug-resistant gram-negative infections.

■ PHARMACOKINETICS AND PHARMACODYNAMICS

- In Elores, ceftriaxone acts to inhibit bacterial cell wall synthesis following attachment to penicillin-binding proteins (PBPs) which inhibits mucopeptide synthesis in the bacterial cell wall leading to bactericidal activity.
- Sulbactam has intrinsic antimicrobial activity for *Acinetobacter baumannii,* and also protects ceftriaxone from degradation by inactivating a broader range of beta-lactamases.
- A synergistic effect is observed when sulbactam is associated with beta-lactam antibiotic that has a complementary affinity for the target sites.
- Elores concentrates in the urine are five to ten times higher than those found in the plasma.

■ AVAILABLE FORMULATIONS

Powder for injection for intravenous (IV) use only

Elores injection 1.5 g; each single dose 1.5-g vial contains ceftriaxone sodium IP equivalent to ceftriaxone (1,000 mg), sulbactam sodium IP equivalent to sulbactam (500 mg), and disodium edetate IP 37 mg.

■ ROUTE OF ADMINISTRATION

Elores is to be administered intravenously after reconstitution over a period of 90 minutes (reduces the chances of thrombophlebitis and other infusion-related reactions).

■ DOSE AND ADMINISTRATION

Neonate: 75–100 mg/kg/day in one to two divided doses

■ CAUTION, PRECAUTIONS, AND RED FLAGS

- Elores is contraindicated in neonates with known hypersensitivity to cephalosporins.
- Ceftriaxone can displace bilirubin from its binding to serum albumin and can predispose to bilirubin encephalopathy.

- Elores must not be mixed or administered simultaneously with any calcium-containing IV solutions, even via different infusion lines or at different infusion sites.

ADVERSE EFFECTS

Localized pain, swelling at injection site, edema, rash

MONITORING

Monitor complete blood count (CBC) weekly, especially in patients receiving Elores for longer than 2 weeks.

Fosfomycin

■ TRADE NAMES

Novefos 8 g sachet, Fosidol powder 8 g, Fosirol sachet 8 g, Monurol 3 g sachet

■ INDICATIONS

- Alternative treatment strategy for empirical management of hospital- or community-acquired multidrug-resistant (MDR) gram-negative sepsis in neonates.
- Fosfomycin is bactericidal and exhibits activity against gram-positive and gram-negative bacteria, including methicillin-resistant *Staphylococcus aureus*, vancomycin-resistant *Enterococcus* spp., extended spectrum beta-lactamase (ESBL) producers, and may penetrate biofilms.

■ PHARMACOKINETICS AND PHARMACODYNAMICS

- Fosfomycin is bactericidal in its effect, targeting mucopeptide synthesis by inhibiting phosphoenolpyruvate transferase, which is the first enzyme involved in peptidoglycan synthesis.
- The intravenous (IV) formulation of fosfomycin (fosfomycin disodium) achieves efficacious concentrations following administration into cerebrospinal fluid, soft tissues, and bone.

■ DOSE AND ADMINISTRATION

- *Premature infants:* 100 mg/kg/day divided into two doses
- *Full-term newborns:* 200 mg/kg/day in three doses

■ CAUTION, PRECAUTIONS, AND RED FLAGS

Contraindicated for use in patients who have known hypersensitivity to fosfomycin.

■ ADVERSE EFFECTS

- Serious side effects include congestive heart failure (3%) due to higher sodium concentration in fosfomycin and hypokalemia (particularly following shorter infusion times).
- It is hypothesized that the body may attempt to compensate for the administered sodium load by increasing renal sodium excretion with concomitant potassium excretion and hypokalemia

■ MONITORING

- Obtain baseline complete blood count (CBC) and kidney function test (KFT)
- Serum electrolytes need to be monitored biweekly

Linezolid

■ TRADE NAMES

Zyvox/Linospan/Linid

■ INDICATIONS

- Limited to treatment of infections caused by gram-positive organisms (methicillin-resistant *Staphylococcus aureus*, penicillin-resistant *Streptococcus pneumoniae*, and vancomycin-resistant *Enterococcus faecium*) that are refractory to conventional therapy with vancomycin and other antibiotics.
- Do not use as empiric treatment.

■ PHARMACOKINETICS AND PHARMACODYNAMICS

- Linezolid is an oxazolidinone agent that has a unique mechanism of inhibition of bacterial protein synthesis.
- It is usually bacteriostatic, although it may be bactericidal against *S. pneumoniae*, *Bacteroides fragilis*, and *Clostridium perfringens*.
- Rapidly penetrates osteoarticular tissues and synovial fluid
- Cerebrospinal fluid (CSF) concentrations were 70% of plasma concentrations in older patients with noninflamed meninges.
- Excreted in the urine as unchanged drug (30%) and two inactive metabolites.
- Serum half-life in most neonates is 2–3 hours, with the exception of preterm neonates <1 week of age, who have a serum half-life of 5–6 hours.

■ AVAILABLE FORMULATIONS

- Linezolid intravenous (IV) injection is supplied as 2-mg/mL solution in single-use, ready-to-use 100-mL, 200-mL, and 300-mL plastic infusion bags in a foil laminate overwrap. IV injection may exhibit a yellow color that can intensify over time without affecting potency.
- An oral suspension is available, and after reconstitution with 123 mL of distilled water (in two portions) provides 20 mg/mL.

■ ROUTE OF ADMINISTRATION

- *Intravenous:* Give as an intermittent IV infusion over 30–120 minutes; supplied as ready-to-use infusion bags (2 mg/mL); no further dilution is necessary.
- *Oral:* May administer without regard to timing of feedings; before administering oral suspension, gently mix by inverting bottle three to five times. Do not shake.

■ DOSE AND ADMINISTRATION

Neonate: <1 kg
- *<14 days old:* 10 mg/kg/dose IV Q12 hours
- *≥14 days old:* 10 mg/kg/dose IV Q8 hours

≥1–2 kg:
- *<7 days old:* 10 mg/kg/dose IV/PO Q12 hours
- *≥7 days old:* 10 mg/kg/dose IV/PO Q8 hours
- *>2 kg:* 10 mg/kg/dose IV/PO Q8 hours

Alternate dosing by gestational age:
<34-week gestation:
- *<7 days old:* 10 mg/kg/dose IV/PO Q12 hours
- *≥7 days old:* 10 mg/kg/dose IV/PO Q8 hours

≥34-week gestation and 0–28 days old: 10 mg/kg/dose IV/PO Q8 hours

■ CAUTION, PRECAUTIONS, AND RED FLAGS

Myelosuppression (including anemia, leukopenia, pancytopenia, and thrombocytopenia) has been reported.

■ ADVERSE EFFECTS

- Elevated transaminases and diarrhea occur in approximately 5% of treated patients; thrombocytopenia and anemia occur in 2%–5%.
- Severe cutaneous adverse reactions such as toxic epidermal necrolysis and Stevens–Johnson syndrome have also been reported.

■ SOLUTION COMPATIBILITY

D5W, normal saline (NS), lactated Ringer's

■ MONITORING

- Monitor complete blood count (CBC) weekly, especially in patients receiving linezolid for longer than 2 weeks.
- Monitor lactate concentrations in patients receiving extended courses of linezolid therapy or in patients with preexisting hepatic or renal dysfunction.

■ FURTHER READING

1. Harriet Service (Johns Hopkins Hospital); Kleinman K, McDaniel L, Molloy M. The Harriet Lane Handbook: A Manual for Pediatric House Officers, 22nd edition. Philadelphia: Elsevier; 2021.
2. Young TE, Magnum B. Micromedex NeoFax Essentials. New Jersey: Thomson Reuters; 2020.

Meropenem

■ TRADE NAMES

Meronem, Merocrit, Meromac

■ INDICATIONS

For sepsis, intraabdominal infections, and meningitis due to gram-negative bacteria

■ PHARMACOKINETICS AND PHARMACODYNAMICS

- It is a broad-spectrum carbapenem antibiotic which penetrates well into the cerebrospinal fluid (CSF) and most body tissues.
- It exhibits the time-dependent killing of gram-negative and gram-positive pathogens.
- Plasma protein binding is minimal.
- Clearance is directly related to renal function, and 70% of a dose is recovered intact in the urine.
- The hepatic function does not affect pharmacokinetics.

■ AVAILABLE FORMULATIONS

Injection: 125 mg, 250 mg, 500 mg and 1-g vials powder forms

■ ROUTE OF ADMINISTRATION

- *Intravenous (IV):* Administer by IV infusion over 30 minutes at a concentration of 1–20 mg/mL
- There is some data that promote prolonged infusions (e.g., over 4 hours) particularly for resistant organisms in neonates.

■ DOSE AND MAXIMUM DOSE

Category	Dose (mg/kg/dose)				
	≤2 kg			>2 kg	
	≤14 days old	15–28 days old	29–60 days old	≤14 days old	15–60 days old
Sepsis					
Meningitis	20 Q12 hourly	20 Q8 hourly	30 Q8 hourly	20 Q8 hourly	30 Q8 hourly

Severe sepsis with moderately resistant meropenem isolate:
>30-week gestation and >7 days old: 40 mg/kg/dose IV Q8 hours

Central nervous system (CNS) infection:
- 40 mg/kg/dose at the recommended age-specific dosing interval

- *<32 weeks gestational age (GA) and <14 days postnatal age (PNA):* Every 12 hours
- *<32 weeks GA and 14 days PNA and older:* Every 8 hours
- *32 weeks GA and older:* Every 8 hours

■ CAUTION, PRECAUTIONS, AND RED FLAGS

- Contraindicated in carbapenem hypersensitivity or previous anaphylactic reactions to beta-lactams.
- Coadministration with valproic acid or divalproex sodium is generally not recommended due to a reduction in valproic acid concentrations that may not respond to a dose increase. If coadministration of meropenem is necessary, supplemental anticonvulsant therapy is recommended.

■ SOLUTION COMPATIBILITY

D5W, D10W, and normal saline (NS)

■ ADVERSE EFFECTS

- *Gastrointestinal tract (GIT):* Diarrhea (4%), nausea/vomiting (1%), and rash (2%), inflammation at the injection site
- The risks of pseudomembranous colitis and fungal infections are also increased.

■ MONITORING

- Complete blood count (CBC) (for thrombocytosis and eosinophilia)
- Liver function test (LFT) for hepatic transaminases
- Assess IV site for signs of inflammation

■ FURTHER READING

1. Harriet Service (Johns Hopkins Hospital); Kleinman K, McDaniel L, Molloy M. The Harriet Lane Handbook: A Manual for Pediatric House Officers, 22nd edition. Philadelphia: Elsevier; 2021.
2. Young TE, Magnum B. Micromedex NeoFax Essentials. New Jersey: Thomson Reuters; 2020.

Piperacillin Tazobactam

■ TRADE NAMES

Zosyn/Tazira/Truzol

■ INDICATIONS

Septicemia and meningitis due to gram-negative organisms

■ PHARMACOKINETICS AND PHARMACODYNAMICS

- Piperacillin/tazobactam combines the extended-spectrum antibiotic piperacillin with the beta-lactamase inhibitor tazobactam.
- Both piperacillin and tazobactam are 30% bound to plasma proteins.
- In noninflamed meninges, the distribution of piperacillin and tazobactam into cerebrospinal fluid (CSF) is low.
- Both piperacillin and tazobactam are eliminated by glomerular filtration and tubular secretion.
- Piperacillin is excreted rapidly as unchanged drug (68% excreted unchanged). Tazobactam and its metabolite are eliminated primarily by renal excretion (80% excreted unchanged).

■ AVAILABLE FORMULATIONS

Injection, powder: 2 g piperacillin and 0.25 g tazobactam; 3 g piperacillin and 0.375 g tazobactam; 4 g piperacillin and 0.5 g tazobactam

■ ROUTE OF ADMINISTRATION

Infuse intravenous (IV) over at least 30 minutes

■ DOSE AND ADMINISTRATION

All doses based on piperacillin component

Based on weight:

Weight	Postnatal	Dose-IV	Interval
<1 kg	0–14 days	100 mg/kg/dose	12 hours
	15–28 days		8 hours
≥1 kg	0–7 days	100 mg/kg/dose	12 hours
	8–28 days		8 hours

Based on gestational age:

Postmenstrual age (PMA) (weeks)	Postnatal	Dose-IV	Interval
29 weeks or less	0–28 days	100 mg/kg/dose	12 hours
	>28 days		8 hours
30–36 weeks	0–14 days	100 mg/kg/dose	12 hours
	>14 days		8 hours
37–44 weeks	0–7 days	100 mg/kg/dose	12 hours
	>7 days		8 hours
>45 weeks	0 to 28 days	100 mg/kg/dose	8 hours

■ CAUTION, PRECAUTIONS, AND RED FLAGS

- Contraindicated in patients with a history of hypersensitivity reactions to any of the penicillins, cephalosporins, or beta-lactamase inhibitors.
- Serious cutaneous reactions [e.g., Stevens–Johnson syndrome, toxic epidermal necrolysis, drug reaction with eosinophilia and systemic symptoms (DRESS)]
- Hypokalemia
- Use caution in neonates requiring sodium restriction as product contains 2.84 mEq (65 mg) of sodium per gram of piperacillin.
- Leukopenia and neutropenia have been reported, especially with prolonged use; usually reversible upon discontinuation; however, monitoring recommended.
- Nephrotoxicity

■ ADVERSE EFFECTS

- Nephrotoxicity
- Rash and hypotension
- Neutropenia ad neutropenia
- Phlebitis

■ SOLUTION COMPATIBILITY

D5W, D10W, normal saline (NS), and lactated Ringer's (LR)

■ MONITORING

- Monitor electrolytes periodically in patients with low potassium reserves.
- Periodic assessment of hematopoietic function, especially with prolonged therapy of 21 days or greater.

■ FURTHER READING

1. Harriet Service (Johns Hopkins Hospital); Kleinman K, McDaniel L, Molloy M. The Harriet Lane Handbook: A Manual for Pediatric House Officers, 22nd edition. Philadelphia: Elsevier; 2021.
2. Young TE, Magnum B. Micromedex NeoFax Essentials. New Jersey: Thomson Reuters; 2020.

Tigecycline

■ TRADE NAMES

Tigez 50 mg injection, Tigi 50 mg injection, Tiganex 50 mg injection, Tigetop 50 mg injection

■ INDICATIONS

- Tigecycline, a derivative of minocycline, is the first drug of the new glycylcycline class of extended-spectrum antibiotics, with a large broad spectrum of in vitro activity.
- Tigecycline has maintained in vitro activity against a wide spectrum of aerobic and anaerobic bacteria which includes methicillin-resistant *Staphylococcus aureus* (MRSA) carbapenem-resistant Enterobacteriaceae (CRE) infections

■ PHARMACOKINETICS AND PHARMACODYNAMICS

- Tigecycline binds reversibly to a helical region (H34) on the 30S subunit of the bacterial ribosome, blocking the binding of transfer RNA to the A site of the ribosome.
- Tigecycline has a high apparent volume of distribution that indicates a high concentration outside vascular space and good penetration in tissues.
- The primary route of tigecycline elimination is biliary excretion, from which the agent emerges unaltered (59%). Secondary routes include renal excretion (22%) and glucuronidation.

■ AVAILABLE FORMULATIONS

Powder for injection for intravenous (IV) use only
   Each single-dose 10-mL glass vial contain 50 mg of tigecycline

■ DOSE AND ADMINISTRATION

- Tigecycline has been used at a dose of 1–1.2 mg/kg every 12 hours (data on neonates limited).
- It is usually administered intravenously over a period of 30 minutes to 1 hour infusion.

■ CAUTION, PRECAUTIONS, AND RED FLAGS

- Contraindicated for use in neonates who have known hypersensitivity to tigecycline.

- Increases in total bilirubin concentration, prothrombin time, and transaminases have been seen in patients treated with tigecycline.

■ ADVERSE EFFECTS

Allergic skin reactions, hepatic failure, anaphylaxis

■ MONITORING

Obtain baseline blood coagulation parameters, including fibrinogen, and continue to monitor regularly during treatment with tigecycline.

Vancomycin

■ TRADE NAMES

Vancocin, Forstaf, Vanlid

■ INDICATIONS

- Drug of choice for serious infections caused by methicillin-resistant staphylococci (*Staphylococcus aureus* and *Staphylococcus epidermidis*) and penicillin-resistant pneumococci
- Gram-positive sepsis
- Ventriculitis-device associated infections

■ PHARMACOKINETICS AND PHARMACODYNAMICS

- Vancomycin is bactericidal for most gram-positive bacteria, but bacteriostatic for enterococci.
- It interferes with cell wall synthesis, inhibits RNA synthesis, and alters plasma membrane function.
- It has poor oral absorption.
- Minimal penetration into the cerebrospinal fluid (CSF) in absence of inflamed meninges.
- Elimination is primarily by glomerular filtration (80%–90% recovered unchanged in urine), with a small amount of hepatic metabolism.
- Mean half-life of 3–4 hours in infants

■ AVAILABLE FORMULATIONS

Injection: 500-mg and 1-g vials

■ ROUTE OF ADMINISTRATION

Intravenous: Administer by intermittent IV infusion over 60–120 minutes (no >10 mg/minute) at a concentration not to exceed 5 mg/mL

■ DOSE AND ADMINISTRATION

Initial dose: 10–15 mg/kg/dose IV every 6–18 hours

Initial dose intervals: Bacteremia: 10 mg/kg/dose, meningitis, pneumonia: 15 mg/kg/dose

Postmenstrual age	Postnatal age	Interval
29 weeks or less	• 0–14 days • Older than 14 days	• 18 hours • 12 hours
30–36 weeks	• 0-14 days • Older than 14 days	• 12 hours • 8 hours
37–44 weeks	• 0–7 days • Older than 7 days	• 12 hours • 8 hours
45 weeks or more	All	6 hours

■ CAUTION, PRECAUTIONS, AND RED FLAGS

- When administered with aminoglycosides, increased risk of nephrotoxicity/ototoxicity
- Extravasation may lead to tissue necrosis.

■ ADVERSE EFFECTS

- Nephrotoxicity and ototoxicity
- Red man syndrome is associated with rapid IV infusion; infuse over 60 minutes (may infuse over 120 minutes if 60-minute infusion is not tolerated). *Note*: Diphenhydramine is used to reverse red man syndrome.
- Neutropenia
- Phlebitis, extravasation may cause tissue necrosis, can be treated with hyaluronidase.

■ MONITORING

- Auditory evaluation
- Renal function tests
- Periodic monitoring of white blood cell count should be done to screen for neutropenia
- Monitor vital signs and blood pressure continuously.

■ FURTHER READING

1. Harriet Service (Johns Hopkins Hospital); Kleinman K, McDaniel L, Molloy M. The Harriet Lane Handbook: A Manual for Pediatric House Officers, 22nd edition. Philadelphia: Elsevier; 2021.
2. Young TE, Magnum B. Micromedex NeoFax Essentials. New Jersey: Thomson Reuters; 2020.

Antiepileptics

Phenobarbital

■ TRADE NAME

Gardenal, Fenobarb, Barbinol, Cenbutal, Appilic

■ INDICATIONS

- One of the first-line drug to control the neonatal seizure; neonatal abstinence syndrome treatment
- May enhance bile excretion in neonatal cholestasis before 99Tc-IDA scanning
- May be considered in prolonged neonatal jaundice

■ PHARMACOKINETICS AND PHARMACODYNAMICS

- Approximately 30% protein-bound
- Primarily metabolized by liver, then excreted in the urine as p-hydroxyphenobarbital which has no anticonvulsant activity; serum half-life in neonates is 40–200 hours.
- The onset of action is within 5 and 20–60 minutes in case of intravenous and oral administration respectively.
- The duration of action is for 4–6 hours after intravenous administration. The enteral preparation is well-absorbed, so transition from parenteral to enteral is good.

■ AVAILABLE FORMULATIONS

Injections: 200 mg/mL (common), 130 mg/mL, 65 mg/mL

Tablet: 30 mg, 60 mg

Syrup: 20 mg/5 mL

■ ROUTE

Intravenous, oral

■ MAXIMUM DOSE

Neonatal seizure: Loading dose is 20 mg/kg diluted to a concentration of 1:10 intravenous followed by 10 mg/kg dose till maximum dose of 40 mg/kg.

Maintenance dose: 3–5 mg/kg/day (up to 8 mg/kg/day) Q12–24 hourly to be started after 12–24 hours of loading dose.

*Intramuscular dose should be 10%–15% higher than intravenous dose.

Neonatal abstinence syndrome:

Loading dose: 16 mg/kg orally on day 1

Maintenance: 1–4 mg/kg/dose orally every 12 hours; weaning is done based on abstinence scoring, by decreasing dose 20% per day.

■ CAUTIONS, PRECAUTIONS, AND RED FLAGS

It can lead to respiratory depression and hypotension, so baby should be watched for need of ventilation and shock.

■ ADMINISTRATION AND EXAMPLE OF PRESCRIPTION

The intravenous administration needs to be slowed over 15–20 minutes. Rate of infusion: 1 mg/kg/min; 30 mg/min maximum.

Dilution: To be diluted in normal saline prior to administration; it is compatible with D5, D10, and normal saline.

For a 3 kg baby loading dose @ 20 mg /kg would be: 20 × 3 mg: 60 mg = 0.3 mL (60/200) phenobarbitone injection to be diluted in 5–10 mL normal saline and given as infusion over 20 minutes.

■ CONTRAINDICATIONS

Marked liver dysfunction

■ ADVERSE EFFECTS

Short-term: Sedation, respiratory depression, hypotension, dilated pupils and doll's eye phenomenon, thrombophlebitis

Long-term: Effect on attention, memory, and cognition

■ MONITORING AND PRECAUTIONS

- Therapeutic blood level is 10–25 µg/mL (neonatal seizure); 20–30 µg/mL (neonatal abstinence syndrome); altered serum concentration may occur with simultaneous administration of other anticonvulsants.
- The intravenous site should be watched for extravasation/ thrombophlebitis.

■ FURTHER READING

1. Harriet Lane Service (Johns Hopkins Hospital); Hughes HK, Kahl LK. Harriet Lane Handbook: A Manual for Pediatric House Officers, 21st edition. St. Louis: Elsevier Health Sciences; 2018.
3. Micormedex NeoFax Essentials 2014. Available from: https://ypeda.com/attachments/fil/Micormedex%20NeoFax%20Essentials%202014%20(1).pdf [Last accessed March, 2024].
2. Volpe JJ. Volpe's Neurology of the Newborn, 6th edition. Philadelphia: WB Saunders Co; 2018.

Phenytoin

■ TRADE NAME

Dilantin, Epsolin, Eptoin, Phenytk, Phalin, Epileptin

■ INDICATIONS

Anticonvulsant drug to control the neonatal seizure

■ PHARMACOKINETICS AND PHARMACODYNAMICS

- Serum half-life is 18–60 hours.
- It has very high (85%–90%) protein binding.
- Hepatic metabolism capacity is limited; saturation may occur within therapeutic range; pharmacokinetics are dose-dependent.
- Elimination rate is increased during first few weeks of life.
- Bilirubin displaces phenytoin from protein-binding sites, resulting in increased serum-free phenytoin concentration.
- The transition to enteral preparation is challenging because of erratic absorption in neonates.
- Onset of action is 30–60 minutes after intravenous (IV) infusion.

■ AVAILABLE FORMULATIONS

Injections: 50 mg/mL, tablet: 50 mg, 100 mg, syrup: 30 mg/5 mL

■ ROUTE

Intravenous, oral (not preferred in neonates)

Loading dose: 15–20 mg/kg IV infusion over at least 30 minutes

Maintenance dose: 4–8 mg/kg/day Q8–12 hourly slow IV infusion

■ CAUTIONS, PRECAUTIONS, AND RED FLAGS

It can lead to hypotension and cardiac arrhythmia.

■ ADMINISTRATION AND EXAMPLE OF PRESCRIPTION

- The intravenous administration should be slow over 15–20 minutes.
- *Maximum rate of infusion:* 0.5–1 mg/kg per minute or 50 mg/min whichever is slower. Intravenous line should be flushed before and after administration.
- Central line should be avoided because of the risk of precipitation.
- Intramuscular (IM) route not acceptable as the drug crystallizes in muscle.
- *Dilution:* To be diluted only in normal saline prior to administration; it is not compatible and is highly unstable with any other solution. It should be used as early as after its preparation.

- For a 3 kg baby loading dose @ 20 mg/kg would be: 20 × 3 mg: 60 mg = 1.2 mL (60/50) of phenytoin injection (1 mL = 50-mg preparation) to be diluted in 10 mL normal saline and given as infusion over 20 minutes.

CONTRAINDICATIONS

Known hypersensitivity to phenytoin and cardiac conduction defects

ADVERSE EFFECTS

Short-term: These include hypotension, cardiac arrhythmia, extravasation, purple glove syndrome (even without extravasation), seizures (at higher concentration), nystagmus, and hypersensitivity reactions.

Long-term: This include gingival hyperplasia, coarsening of the facies, hirsutism, hyperglycemia, and drug-induced lupus.

MONITORING AND PRECAUTIONS

- The baby should be monitored for electrocardiogram (ECG), blood pressure, and respiratory function during and up to 1 hour after infusion.
- Therapeutic blood level is 6–15 µg/mL in the first weeks and 10–20 µg/mL later. Trough level should be taken for monitoring.
- Altered serum concentration may occur with simultaneous administration of drugs, i.e., carbamazepine, cimetidine, corticosteroids, digoxin, furosemide, phenobarbital, and valproate due to drug interaction.
- The IV site should be watched for extravasation/thrombophlebitis.

FURTHER READING

1. Harriet Lane Service (Johns Hopkins Hospital); Hughes HK, Kahl LK. Harriet Lane Handbook: A Manual for Pediatric House Officers, 21st edition. St. Louis: Elsevier Health Sciences; 2018.
2. Micormedex NeoFax Essentials 2014. Available from: https://ypeda.com/attachments/fil/Micormedex%20NeoFax%20Essentials%202014%20(1).pdf [Last accessed March, 2024].
3. Volpe JJ. Volpe's Neurology of the Newborn, 6th edition. Philadelphia: WB Saunders Co; 2018.

Fosphenytoin

■ TRADE NAME

Fosentin, Fosolin, Fosphen

■ INDICATIONS

Anticonvulsant drug to control the neonatal seizure

■ PHARMACOKINETICS AND PHARMACODYNAMICS

- Fosphenytoin is a water-soluble prodrug of phenytoin rapidly converted by phosphatases in blood and tissue.
- Its pharmacologic activity is only after conversion to phenytoin.
- Each 1.5 mg of fosphenytoin is metabolically converted to 1 mg of phenytoin.
- The peak concentration reaches 20–30 minutes after intravenous administration.
- Conversion half-life of fosphenytoin is approximately 8 minutes.
- Fosphenytoin is highly protein bound (95%–99%). Its primary elimination is by hepatic metabolism.
- Renal excretion is negligible.
- Serum half-life (18–70 hours) is that of same as reflects that of phenytoin.
- Fosphenytoin has neutral pH as compared to that of basic pH of phenytoin.

■ AVAILABLE FORMULATIONS

Injections: 75 mg (50 mg PE)/mL fosphenytoin dosing is expressed in phenytoin equivalents (PE) (fosphenytoin 1 mg PE = phenytoin 1 mg).

■ ROUTE

Intravenous (IV), intramuscular (IM)

■ MAXIMUM DOSE

Loading dose: 15–20 mg PE/kg IM or IV infusion over 10–20 minutes

Maintenance dose: 4–8 mg PE/kg/day Q 12 hourly IM or IV 24 hours after loading dose

■ CAUTIONS, PRECAUTIONS, AND RED FLAGS

It can lead to hypotension and cardiac arrhythmia.

■ ADMINISTRATION AND EXAMPLE OF PRESCRIPTION

- The intravenous infusion should be at a rate of 1–3 mg PE/kg/min (maximum 150 mg PE/min) at a concentration of 1.5–25 mg PE/mL.
- It can be diluted in 5% dextrose or normal saline and can be administered at faster rate.
- The risk of extravasation is lesser as compared to that of phenytoin.
- Intramuscular administration can be undiluted. It may be given in divided doses at more than one site.
- For a 3 kg baby loading dose @ 20 mg PE/kg would be: 20 × 3 mg: 60 mg = 1.2 mL (60/50) fosphenytoin injection to be diluted in 10 mL normal saline and given as infusion over 20 minutes.

■ CONTRAINDICATIONS

Known hypersensitivity to phenytoin cardiac conduction defects

■ ADVERSE EFFECTS

Side effect profile is same as phenytoin but to lesser extent.

■ MONITORING AND PRECAUTIONS

- The baby should be monitored for electrocardiogram (ECG), blood pressure, and respiratory function during and up to 1 hour after infusion.
- Therapeutic blood level 10–20 µg/mL.
- The intravenous site should be watched for extravasation/thrombophlebitis.

■ FURTHER READING

1. Harriet Lane Service (Johns Hopkins Hospital); Hughes HK, Kahl LK. Harriet Lane Handbook: A Manual for Pediatric House Officers, 21st edition. St. Louis: Elsevier Health Sciences; 2018.
2. Micormedex NeoFax Essentials 2014. Available from: https://ypeda.com/attachments/fil/Micormedex%20NeoFax%20Essentials%202014%20(1).pdf [Last accessed March, 2024].
3. Volpe JJ. Volpe's Neurology of the Newborn, 6th edition. Philadelphia: WB Saunders Co; 2018.

Midazolam

■ TRADE NAME

Mezolam, Midaver, Midoryx, Fulsed Midacip, Insed (nasal spray)

■ INDICATIONS

- Anticonvulsant drug to control the neonatal seizure
- For sedation

■ PHARMACOKINETICS AND PHARMACODYNAMICS

- Midazolam is short-acting benzodiazepine with rapid onset of action.
- It is metabolized by hepatic CYP3A4 to a less active hydroxylated metabolite.
- The excretion is renal.
- It is highly protein-bound.
- The duration of action is 2–6 hours.
- Elimination half-life is variable (approximately 4–6 hours in term neonates, and up to 22 hours in premature babies).
- Bioavailability is 50% with sublingual/intranasal administration and 36% with oral administration.

■ AVAILABLE FORMULATIONS

Injections: 1 mg/mL, 5 mg/mL, 0.5 mg per puff in nasal spray

Tablet: 7.5 mg, 15 mg

Syrup: 2 mg/mL

■ ROUTE

Intravenous, intramuscular, intranasal, sublingual, oral

■ MAXIMUM DOSE

For seizures: 0.2 mg/kg intravenous over 10 minutes followed by 0.1–0.4 mg/kg/h

For sedation: 0.05–0.15 mg/kg intravenous over at least 5 minutes; repeat as required, usually every 2–4 hours.

Intranasal dose: 0.2 mg/kg

Sublingual dose: 0.2 mg/kg

Oral: 0.25 mg/kg per dose

■ CAUTIONS, PRECAUTIONS, AND RED FLAGS

It can lead to hypotension and respiratory depression. Paradoxical seizures have also been reported.

■ ADMINISTRATION AND EXAMPLE OF PRESCRIPTION

Midazolam is compatible with normal saline, dextrose, and sterile water for injection. For a 3 kg baby loading dose @ 0.2 mg/kg would be: 0.2×3 mg = 0.6 mg = 0.6 mL [(0.6/1) of 1 mg/mL preparation] midazolam injection to be diluted in 5 mL normal saline and given over 10 minutes.

Maintenance: @ 0.1 mg/kg/h =$0.1 \times 3 \times 24 = 7.2$ mg. So, for maintenance 7.2 mL of 1 mg/mL, midazolam preparation should be diluted in normal saline up to 15 mL and to be set for infusion over 24 hours i.e., @ 0.6 mL/h (15/24).

■ CONTRAINDICATIONS

It should be avoided in case of hypotension and shock.

■ ADVERSE EFFECTS

Respiratory depression, apnea, and hypotension with intravenous use; burning sensation has been reported with intravenous use.

■ MONITORING AND PRECAUTIONS

During intravenous infusion respiratory status and blood pressure should be closely monitored. Liver function should also be assessed. Withdrawal signs may occur after prolonged infusion, therefore slow weaning should be done before discontinuation in case of prolonged therapy.

■ FURTHER READING

1. Harriet Lane Service (Johns Hopkins Hospital); Hughes HK, Kahl LK. Harriet Lane Handbook: A Manual for Pediatric House Officers, 21st edition. St. Louis: Elsevier Health Sciences; 2018.
2. Lingamchetty TN, Hosseini SA, Saadabadi A. Midazolam. In: StatPearls [Internet]. Treasure Island (FL): StatPearls Publishing; 2024.
3. Micormedex NeoFax Essentials 2014. Available from: https://ypeda.com/attachments/fil/Micormedex%20NeoFax%20Essentials%202014%20(1).pdf [Last accessed March, 2024].
4. Volpe JJ. Volpe's Neurology of the Newborn, 6th edition. Philadelphia: WB Saunders Co; 2018.

Lorazepam

■ TRADE NAME

Lopez, Ativan, Lorel, Loricon

■ INDICATIONS

- Anticonvulsant drug to control the neonatal seizure
- For sedation

■ PHARMACOKINETICS AND PHARMACODYNAMICS

- Onset of action within 1–3 minutes, if administered IV, and 15–30 minutes, if administered IM.
- The peak serum concentration reaches within 45 minutes.
- Duration of action is 3–24 hours.
- Mean half-life in term neonates is 40 hours.
- The metabolism to inactive glucuronide occurs in liver and excretion occurs in kidneys.

■ AVAILABLE FORMULATIONS

Injections: 2 mg/mL, 4 mg/mL

Tablet: 2 mg

■ ROUTE

Intravenous (IV), intramuscular, oral

■ MAXIMUM DOSE

0.05–0.1 mg/kg per dose IV slow push over 2–3 minutes

■ CAUTIONS, PRECAUTIONS, AND RED FLAGS

It can lead to respiratory depression. The myoclonic jerks have been reported in premature neonates.

■ ADMINISTRATION AND EXAMPLE OF PRESCRIPTION

Lorazepam is compatible with normal saline, dextrose, and sterile water for injection. For a 3 kg baby loading dose @ 0.1 mg /kg would be: 0.1 × 3 mg = 0.3 mg = 0.15 mL [(0.3/2) of 2 mg/mL preparation] lorazepam injection to be diluted in 5 mL normal saline and given over 3 minutes.

■ CONTRAINDICATIONS

It should be avoided in case of hypotension and shock; known hypersensitivity to lorazepam

■ ADVERSE EFFECTS

Respiratory depression, hypotension, apnea, bradycardia

■ MONITORING AND PRECAUTIONS

Monitoring for respiratory status is needed. Intravenous site should be looked for extravasation.

■ FURTHER READING

1. Ghiasi N, Bhansali RK, Marwaha R. Lorazepam. In: StatPearls. Treasure Island (FL): StatPearls Publishing; 2024.
2. Harriet Lane Service (Johns Hopkins Hospital); Hughes HK, Kahl LK. Harriet Lane Handbook: A Manual for Pediatric House Officers, 21st edition. St. Louis: Elsevier Health Sciences; 2018.
3. Micormedex NeoFax Essentials 2014. Available from: https://ypeda.com/attachments/fil/Micormedex%20NeoFax%20Essentials%202014%20(1).pdf [Last accessed March, 2024].
4. Volpe JJ. Volpe's Neurology of the Newborn, 6th edition. Philadelphia: WB Saunders Co; 2018.

Diazepam

■ TRADE NAME

Valium, Calmpose, Alpazepam, Anxol

■ INDICATIONS

Anticonvulsant drug to control the seizure (not very frequently used in neonates)

■ PHARMACOKINETICS AND PHARMACODYNAMICS

When administered intravenously, diazepam has an onset of action within 1–3 minutes. It has a very rapid clearance, so it is a poor drug for maintenance. The therapeutic dose is variable and is in very narrow range.

■ AVAILABLE FORMULATIONS

Injections: 5 mg/mL, tablet: 2 mg, 5 mg, 10 mg

■ ROUTE

Intravenous (IV), intramuscular oral, rectal

■ MAXIMUM DOSE

0.2–0.75 mg/kg slow IV push

Rectal dose: 0.5–1.0 mg/kg

■ CAUTIONS, PRECAUTIONS, AND RED FLAGS

- It can lead to respiratory depression, hypotension, and apnea.
- When administered with barbiturate, it carries an increased risk of severe circulatory collapse with respiratory failure.
- In many preparations the vehicle for IV diazepam is sodium benzoate, which can increase free bilirubin by displacing it from albumin-binding site and thereby increasing the risk of kernicterus.

■ ADMINISTRATION AND EXAMPLE OF PRESCRIPTION

Lorazepam is compatible with normal saline, dextrose, and sterile water for injection. For a 3 kg baby a dose @ 0.3 mg/kg would be: 0.3×3 mg = 0.9 mg = 0.2 mL [(0.9/5) of 5 mg/mL preparation] diazepam injection to be diluted in 5 mL normal saline and given over 5 minutes.

◼ CONTRAINDICATIONS

It should be avoided in case of hypotension and shock; known hypersensitivity to diazepam

◼ ADVERSE EFFECTS

Respiratory depression, hypotension, apnea, bradycardia, phlebitis

◼ MONITORING AND PRECAUTIONS

Monitoring for respiratory status is needed. IV site should be looked for extravasation.

◼ FURTHER READING

1. Dhaliwal JS, Rosani A, Saadabadi A. Diazepam. In: StatPearls [Internet]. Treasure Island (FL): StatPearls Publishing; 2024.
2. Harriet Lane Service (Johns Hopkins Hospital); Hughes HK, Kahl LK. Harriet Lane Handbook: A Manual for Pediatric House Officers, 21st edition. St. Louis: Elsevier Health Sciences; 2018.
3. Volpe JJ. Volpe's Neurology of the Newborn, 6th edition. Philadelphia: WB Saunders Co; 2018.

Valproic Acid

■ TRADE NAMES

Valparin, ValpreX, Encorate, Epival

■ INDICATIONS

Anticonvulsant drug occasionally used to control seizure in neonates in refractory cases.

■ PHARMACOKINETICS AND PHARMACODYNAMICS

The reported effective therapeutic range for plasma valproic acid levels is 40–100 mg/L (278–694 µmol/L). In patients with severe renal insufficiency, it may be necessary to alter dosage as per plasma levels. The half-life is 8–20 hours. In neonate and young infants, the clearance of valproate is decreased and there is considerable variability in half-life ranging from 1 to 67 hours.

The mechanism of action is by increasing GABA (gamma aminobutyric acid) levels, blocking voltage-gated ion channels, and inhibiting histone deacetylase.

■ AVAILABLE FORMULATIONS

Injections: 100 mg/mL

Syrup: 200 mg/5 mL

Tablet: 200 mg, 300 mg, 500 mg

■ ROUTE

Intravenous, oral

■ MAXIMUM DOSE

The dose is 20–25 mg/kg/day followed by 5–10 mg/kg every 12 hours.

■ CAUTIONS, PRECAUTIONS, AND RED FLAGS

- It can lead to hepatotoxicity, hyperammonemia, transaminitis, and encephalopathy-like illness in babies <2 years of age.
- It should not be used with salicylates in <2 years of age because of increased risk of hepatotoxicity.

■ ADMINISTRATION AND EXAMPLE OF PRESCRIPTION

- Sodium valproate injection can be given by direct slow intravenous injection or by infusion using a separate intravenous line in normal saline, dextrose 5%, or dextrose saline. The intravenous preparation should be administered over 60 minutes infusion.

- Sodium valproate injection should be replaced by oral valproate therapy as soon as practicable. The dosing recommendation remain same both oral as well as intravenous preparation.
- For a 3 kg baby loading dose @ 25 mg /kg would be: 25 × 3 mg: 75 mg = 0.75 mL (75/100) valproic acid injection to be diluted in 10 mL normal saline and given as infusion over 60 minutes.

CONTRAINDICATIONS

- Liver dysfunction
- Family history of hepatic dysfunction urea cycle disorder
- Porphyria mitochondrial disorders

ADVERSE EFFECTS

Hepatotoxicity, elevated blood ammonia levels, thrombo-cytopenia

MONITORING AND PRECAUTIONS

- The baby should be monitored for liver dysfunction.
- The interchange of brand should be avoided.
- It can interact with enzyme inducing drugs, so drug level monitoring become important.

FURTHER READING

1. Alfonso I, Alvarez LA, Gilman J, Dunoyer C, Yelin K, Papazian O. Intravenous valproate dosing in neonates. J Child Neurol. 2000;15(12):827-9.
2. Harriet Lane Service (Johns Hopkins Hospital); Hughes HK, Kahl LK. Harriet Lane Handbook: A Manual for Pediatric House Officers, 21st edition. St. Louis: Elsevier Health Sciences; 2018.
3. Rahman M, Nguyen H. Valproic Acid. In: StatPearls [Internet]. Treasure Island (FL): StatPearls Publishing; 2024.

Levetiracetam

■ TRADE NAME

Levepil, Keppra, Levesam, Levepsy, Levroxa

■ INDICATIONS

Anticonvulsant drug to control the neonatal seizure.

■ PHARMACOKINETICS AND PHARMACODYNAMICS

- Levetiracetam is rapidly absorbed and has very high (96%) bioavailability.
- Peak plasma concentration is achieved in 5–15 minutes with intravenous (IV) use and 60 minutes after oral administration.
- <10% of the drug is protein-bound.
- It is not extensively metabolized, and almost 66% is excreted unchanged by kidneys.
- The plasma half-life in the immediate neonatal period is approximately 18 hours. Dose adjustment is needed in renal impairment.
- There are no known significant drug interactions.

■ AVAILABLE FORMULATIONS

Injections: 100 mg/mL

Syrup: 100 mg/mL

Tablet: 250 mg, 500 mg

■ ROUTE

Intravenous, oral

■ MAXIMUM DOSE

Loading dose is 30–60 mg/kg IV over 30 minutes (total IV loading doses of about 80–100 mg/kg, if needed).

Maintenance dose: 40–60 mg/kg/day in Q8–12 hourly

■ CAUTIONS, PRECAUTIONS, AND RED FLAGS

Dose adjustment may be needed in case of renal impairment.

■ ADMINISTRATION AND EXAMPLE OF PRESCRIPTION

Intravenous: The injection should be diluted to a concentration of 5–15 mg/mL and infused over 15 minutes. Levetiracetam is compatible with normal saline, dextrose, and sterile water for injection. For a 3 kg baby a loading dose @ 40 mg/kg would be: 40×3 mg = 120 mg = 1.2 mL [(120/100) of 100 mg/mL preparation] levetiracetam injection to be diluted in 10 mL normal saline and given over 15 minutes.

■ CONTRAINDICATIONS

Known hypersensitivity to levetiracetam

■ ADVERSE EFFECTS

It is mostly safe. Sedation and irritability have been reported in a few cases.

■ MONITORING AND PRECAUTIONS

- It has a wide therapeutic index. The drug level monitoring is not required.
- Therapeutic concentrations are approximately 10–40 µg/mL.

■ FURTHER READING

1. Harriet Lane Service (Johns Hopkins Hospital); Hughes HK, Kahl LK. Harriet Lane Handbook: A Manual for Pediatric House Officers, 21st edition. St. Louis: Elsevier Health Sciences; 2018.
2. Kumar A, Maini K, Kadian R. Levetiracetam. In: StatPearls. Treasure Island (FL): StatPearls Publishing; 2024.
3. Micormedex NeoFax Essentials 2014. Available from: https://ypeda.com/attachments/fil/Micormedex%20NeoFax%20Essentials%202014%20(1).pdf [Last accessed March, 2024].
4. Volpe JJ. Volpe's Neurology of the Newborn, 6th edition. Philadelphia: WB Saunders Co; 2018.

Lidocaine

■ TRADE NAME

Lignocin, Lidocare

■ INDICATIONS

Anticonvulsant drug to control the neonatal seizure

■ PHARMACOKINETICS AND PHARMACODYNAMICS

- Onset of action is 1–2 minutes after bolus administration.
- Plasma half-life in neonates is 3 hours.
- Metabolism occurs in the liver and approximately 30% is excreted unchanged in neonates.

■ AVAILABLE FORMULATIONS

Injections: 10 mg/mL (1%), 20 mg/mL (2%)

■ ROUTE

Intravenous

■ MAXIMUM DOSE

Loading dose of 2 mg/kg in 10 minutes, followed by a continuous infusion of 6 mg/kg/h for 6 hours, then 4 mg/kg/h for 12 hours, followed by 2 mg/kg/h for 12 hours.

■ CAUTIONS, PRECAUTIONS, AND RED FLAGS

It should not be administered with phenytoin due to risk of cumulative cardiac toxicity. Lidocaine dose should be adjusted during therapeutic hypothermia because of decreased clearance. Reduced dose is needed in premature babies. It should not be used for more than 36 hours because of cumulative risk of toxicity.

■ ADMINISTRATION AND EXAMPLE OF PRESCRIPTION

Intravenous: The lidocaine injection is compatible with dextrose and normal saline.

For a 3 kg baby a loading dose @ 2 mg/kg would be: 2 × 3 mg = 6 mg = 0.6 mL [(6/10) of 10 mg/mL preparation] lidocaine injection to be diluted in 10 mL normal saline and given over 10 minutes. The maintenance infusion @ 6 mg/kg/h for next 6 hours would be: 6 × 3 mg = 18 mg = 1.8 mL [(18/10) of 10 mg/mL preparation] to be diluted in 15 mL normal saline and given @ 2.5 mL/h (15/6) for next 6 hours

■ CONTRAINDICATIONS

Congenital heart disease, complete heart block, and wide complex tachycardia

■ ADVERSE EFFECTS

Arrhythmia (ventricular tachycardia), hypotension, seizure

■ MONITORING AND PRECAUTIONS

- The baby should be under electrocardiogram (ECG) monitoring for detection of arrhythmia.
- Level >9 mg/L is toxic.

■ FURTHER READING

1. Carin MA, Rademaker, de Vries LS. Pharmacology Review: Lidocaine for Neonatal Seizure Management. Neoreviews. December 2008;9(12): e585-e589.
2. Harriet Lane Service (Johns Hopkins Hospital); Hughes HK, Kahl LK. Harriet Lane Handbook: A Manual for Pediatric House Officers, 21st edition. St. Louis: Elsevier Health Sciences; 2018.
3. Micormedex NeoFax Essentials 2014. Available from: https://ypeda.com/attachments/fil/Micormedex%20NeoFax%20Essentials%202014%20(1).pdf [Last accessed March, 2024].
4. Volpe JJ. Volpe's Neurology of the Newborn, 6th edition. Philadelphia: WB Saunders Co; 2018.

Paraldehyde

■ TRADE NAME

Paral

■ INDICATIONS

- Anticonvulsant drug to control the neonatal seizure
- Sedative

■ PHARMACOKINETICS AND PHARMACODYNAMICS

Paraldehyde is rapidly absorbed when administered by oral, rectal, or parenteral route, but is irritating to soft tissue. The reported half-life is 4–10 hours. It has significant elimination by pulmonary route (70%–80%). The exact mechanism of action of paraldehyde is unclear, though it may depress the reticular activating system.

■ AVAILABLE FORMULATIONS

Injections: Paraldehyde injection (100%); 1 g/mL

■ ROUTE

Intravenous, intramuscular, per rectal

■ MAXIMUM DOSE

0.3 mL/kg/dose per rectal
    0.1–0.2 mL/kg intramuscular/200–400 mg/kg deep intramuscular 150 mg/kg/h for 3 hours.

■ CAUTIONS, PRECAUTIONS, AND RED FLAGS

- It should be used with caution in neonates with respiratory distress, as it has been reported to produce pulmonary edema, pulmonary hemorrhage, and hypotension after intravenous administration in older children.
- If possible, all glass syringes should be used with paraldehyde, although, for immediate administration, the drug may be used with a plastic syringe.
- Intra-arterial administration in one case caused generalized arterial and venous thrombosis. Concomitant administration with other central nervous system (CNS) depressants should be avoided.
- The injection should be kept in cool place and protected from light.

ADMINISTRATION AND EXAMPLE OF PRESCRIPTION

- For per rectal use the drug should be mixed in coconut oil in 3:1 ratio. For a baby weighing 3 kg the intramuscular (IM) dose @ 0.2 mL/kg would be: 0.2 × 3 = 0.6 Ml
- For intravenous preparation the drug should be diluted in normal saline. For a baby weighing 3 kg the IM dose @ 150 mg/kg/h for 3 hours would be: 3 × 150 × 3 mg = 1,350 mg = 1.35 mL (1,350/1,000) of 1 g/mL paraldehyde injection. The dose (1.3 mL) should be diluted in 10 mL normal saline and given over 3 hours.

CONTRAINDICATIONS

Severe hepatic dysfunction, severe respiratory compromise

ADVERSE EFFECTS

Pulmonary hemorrhage, pulmonary edema, hypotension, and liver injury

MONITORING AND PRECAUTIONS

Therapeutic serum level is >10 mg/dL. The baby should be monitored for shock and respiratory deterioration.

FURTHER READING

1. Curless RG, Holzman BH, Ramsay RE. Paraldehyde therapy in childhood status epilepticus. Arch Neurol. 1983;40(8):477-80.
2. Koren G, Butt W, Rajchgot P, Mayer J, Whyte H, Pape K, et al. Intravenous paraldehyde for seizure control in newborn infants. Neurology. 1986;36(1):108-11.
3. Mishra D, Gupta VK. Use of paraldehyde in neonates—an experience. Indian Pediatr. 2001;38:209-10.
4. Tulloch JK, Carr RR, Ensom MH. A systematic review of the pharmacokinetics of antiepileptic drugs in neonates with refractory seizures. J Pediatr Pharmacol Ther. 2012;17(1):31-44.
4. Volpe JJ. Volpe's Neurology of the Newborn, 6th edition. Philadelphia: WB Saunders Co; 2018.
6. Wait RB, Greenhalgh D, Gamelli RL. Vascular injury in the neonate associated with intra-arterial injection of paraldehyde. Clin Pediatr (Phila). 1984;23(6):324.

Topiramate

■ TRADE NAME

Topamed, Topirol, Topaz

■ INDICATIONS

- Anticonvulsant drug used as add on therapy to control the neonatal seizure
- Adjunct with hypothermia for neuroprotection

■ PHARMACOKINETICS AND PHARMACODYNAMICS

- Topiramate is rapidly well-absorbed from the gut and is excreted unchanged in urine. It is well-tolerated and has a linear dose–serum concentration response.
- The clearance is prolonged in infants who were undergoing therapeutic hypothermia and in those receiving other anticonvulsants.
- The therapeutic concentrations is 5–20 µg/mL.
- Reported half-life is 35.6 ± 19.3 hours.

■ AVAILABLE FORMULATIONS

Tablet: 25 mg, 50 mg

■ ROUTE

Oral

■ MAXIMUM DOSE

Dose: 3–10 mg/kg/ day in two divided (maximum up to 25 mg/kg/day)

It should be started at 1–3 mg/kg/day as a single dose for the first week. Weekly increment is done by 1–3 mg/kg/day to the recommended total daily dose of 5–10 mg/kg/day in one to two divided doses. The daily dosage should be given as two divided doses.

■ CAUTIONS, PRECAUTIONS, AND RED FLAGS

- The drug should be used with caution in conditions which predisposes to metabolic acidosis. It should be gradually weaned.
- Hyperammonemia with or without encephalopathy may occur with topiramate with or without concomitant valproic acid.

ADMINISTRATION AND EXAMPLE OF PRESCRIPTION

- The tablet should be dissolved in water and required dose is given via orogastric tube. Use mixture immediately. Do not store dissolved tablet for future use.
- The dose @ 6 mg/kg maintenance for 3 kg baby would be: as 3 × 6 = 18 mg/day = 9 mg twice a day. Dissolve 50 mg tablet in 10 mL water and give 1.8 mL (9/50 × 10–1.8 mL) of dissolved solution for one dose.

CONTRAINDICATIONS

Hypersensitivity to any component of the product

ADVERSE EFFECTS

Hyperthermia, hyperammonemia, metabolic acidosis, poor weight gain

MONITORING AND PRECAUTIONS

- Monitor for hyperthermia, metabolic acidosis, ammonia levels, and seizures (if rapid withdrawal of topiramate is needed)
- Monitor renal function, serum bicarbonate, and for metabolic acidosis at baseline and periodically during treatment.
- Ammonia concentration in any infant with lethargy or vomiting

FURTHER READING

1. Donovan MD, Griffin BT, Kharoshankaya L, Cryan JF, Boylan GB. Pharmacotherapy for Neonatal Seizures: Current Knowledge and Future Perspectives. Drugs. 2016;76:647-61.
2. Glass HC, Poulin C, Shevell MI. Topiramate for the treatment of neonatal seizures. Pediatr Neurol. 2011;44(6):439-42.
3. Micormedex NeoFax Essentials 2014. Available from: https://ypeda.com/attachments/fil/Micormedex%20NeoFax%20Essentials%202014%20(1).pdf [Last accessed March, 2024].
4. Volpe JJ. Volpe's Neurology of the Newborn, 6th edition. Philadelphia: WB Saunders Co; 2018.

Pyridoxine

■ TRADE NAME

B star B long, B Six, Ingavit B6, Pyrinate (tablet)

■ INDICATIONS

Diagnosis and treatment of pyridoxine-dependent seizures

■ PHARMACOKINETICS AND PHARMACODYNAMICS

- Its half-life is approximately 15–20 days.
- Vitamin B6 is degraded to 4-pyridoxic acid in the liver
- This metabolite is excreted in the urine.
- Pyridoxine is required for the synthesis of the inhibitory neurotransmitter gamma-aminobutyric acid (GABA). Pyridoxine-dependent seizures are a result of defective binding of pyridoxine in the formation of GABA.

■ AVAILABLE FORMULATIONS

Injection: 100 mg/mL tablet: 10 mg

■ ROUTE

Intravenous (IV), intramuscular (IM), oral

■ MAXIMUM DOSE

Initial diagnostic dose: 50–100 mg IV push or IM; 100 mg dose needs to be repeated every 10 minutes till seizure is controlled or to maximum of 500 mg.

Maintenance dose: 50–100 mg orally every 24 hours; high doses may be required during periods of intercurrent illness.

■ CAUTIONS, PRECAUTIONS, AND RED FLAGS

- Pyridoxine injection contains aluminum that may be toxic with prolonged IV administration in patients with renal impairment or in premature infants (immature kidney function).
- It can result in apnea, bradycardia, or hypotension.

■ ADMINISTRATION AND EXAMPLE OF PRESCRIPTION

- If intravenous preparation is not available, intramuscular route may have to be used (1 mL of injection neurobion has 50 mg pyridoxine and 1 mL each may be administered at two sites).
- Some infants not responsive to pyridoxine may require pyridoxal-5-phosphate (PLP), the active form of vitamin B6. In general, a dose of

50–100 mg/kg divided six times per day is administered for at least a 3- to 5-day trial.
- PLP is only available in enteral forms and has side effects similar to pyridoxine.

CONTRAINDICATIONS

Hypervitaminosis B6, evidence of sensitivity to pyridoxine or to any of the ingredients in pyridoxine hydrochloride injection.

ADVERSE EFFECTS

Hypotension, apnea, neurologic depression

MONITORING AND PRECAUTIONS

Initial administration of pyridoxine should be accompanied by electroencephalogram (EEG) monitoring. Monitor for cardiorespiratory depression. A pyridoxine level <20 nanomoles/L is indicative of deficiency.

FURTHER READING

1. Abosamak NER, Gupta V. Vitamin B6 (Pyridoxine). In: StatPearls. Treasure Island (FL): StatPearls Publishing; 2024.
2. Micormedex NeoFax Essentials 2014. Available from: https://ypeda.com/attachments/fil/Micormedex%20NeoFax%20Essentials%202014%20(1).pdf [Last accessed March, 2024].
3. Surtees R, Wolf N. Treatable neonatal epilepsy. Arch Dis Child. 2007;92(8):659-61.
4. Volpe JJ: Volpe's Neurology of the Newborn, 6th edition. Philadelphia: WB Saunders Co; 2018.

Prevention of Medication Errors

■ DEFINITION OF MEDICATION ERRORS

Medication errors are preventable events that can occur at any time point from ordering the medication, copying the order, dispensing the medicine from pharmacy, preparation, or administration that can lead to patient harm. Some of these errors can cause little impact while others can lead to life-threatening consequences.

■ WHY ARE NEONATES MORE PRONE TO MEDICATION ERRORS?

Physiology: Small body size, physiological immaturity of organs, rapid changes in weight and body surface area

Process- and system-related: Displaced identity bands from wrist or ankles and barriers in communication with the caregivers. Under staffing in SNCU/NICU (special newborn care unit/neonatal intensive care unit), high workload, poor handoffs and communication among health care providers, inappropriate use of technology, inadequate training, and lack of supportive environment to report and rectify medication errors.

■ WHAT ARE THE TYPES OF MEDICATION ERRORS COMMONLY ENCOUNTERED IN THE NICU?

Type of error	Examples
Prescription error	• Wrong drug • Wrong route • Wrong use of units • Wrong weight, dosage regimen • Drug dosage not adjusted to patient characteristics such as renal or hepatic impairment • Dose not adjusted for postnatal age or gestation
Transcription errors	• Illegible handwriting • Patient details not noted in the prescription chart (current weight, day of antibiotic) • Wrong dose due to misplacement of decimals

Contd…

Contd…

Type of error	Examples
Dispensing and administration errors	• Incorrect calculation or preparation in the pharmacy • Late dispensing of medications • Incorrect labeling or dilution of preparation • Patient misidentification • Additional dose of drug • Wrong dilution or diluent or rate of administration • Precautions not taken (for example to protect drug from light) during administration • Mixing with incompatible medications

◼ HOW TO PREVENT MEDICATION ERRORS?

Preventing prescription and transcription errors:

- *Use of a unified local neonatal formulary:* Encourage the use of a standardized formulary in the NICU that contains information for each drug and dosage recommendations. It should also contain information on drug preparation, administration, and storage of diluted preparations. Let dosage book be easily available and accessible in the NICU.
- *Computerized physician order entry (CPOE):* Prescription can be made using computers with built in dosage recommendations, order sets, stop orders, and auto reminders.
- Avoid verbal instructions in drug prescription unless in emergency situations. Even if verbal orders are taken, closed loop communication to be maintained.
- Identify and rectify human factors that result in errors.
  - Review information about patient before prescribing medicines
  - Stress on correct expression of measurement unit (microgram or milligram rather than µg or mg) and decimal placement
    - 0.05 milligram is correct while .05 milligram is incorrect
    - 5 milligram is correct while 5.0 milligram is incorrect
  - If a medication needs specific preparation, then physicians should add those instructions in prescription chart. For example, dilute 20 milligram of phenytoin in 20 mL normal saline and infuse for over 30 minutes.
  - Utilize computers to provide printed prescription to avoid difficult-to-read handwritten physician orders.
  - Nurses normally intervene at the end of the pharmacotherapy process, preparing, and administering drugs. However, they play an important role in detecting errors during the prescribing step by verifying if the medication is for the right indication and double-checking the formulary for dosage and preparation instructions.

Prevention of drug dispensing errors:

- To avoid drug dispensing errors, medications should be labeled and stored properly **(Fig. 1)**.
- Look-alike and soundalike medicines should be stored separately and labeled properly **(Fig. 2)**.
  Soundalike medicines should be labeled properly and stored separately with an alert label. Ideally, they should occupy the opposite corners of a crash cart tray and not be closer together **(Fig. 3)**.
- Use one formulation of a particular drug in the hospital. Minimize the availability of multiple drug strengths. Injection vitamin K is available as 1 mg per 0.5 mL and as 10 mg per 1 mL. Only one formulation should be available for use in the unit.
- Label medications with both generic and trade names to make them easier to distinguish.
- Use additional warning labels to alert staff especially drugs those with serious side effects **(Fig. 4)**.

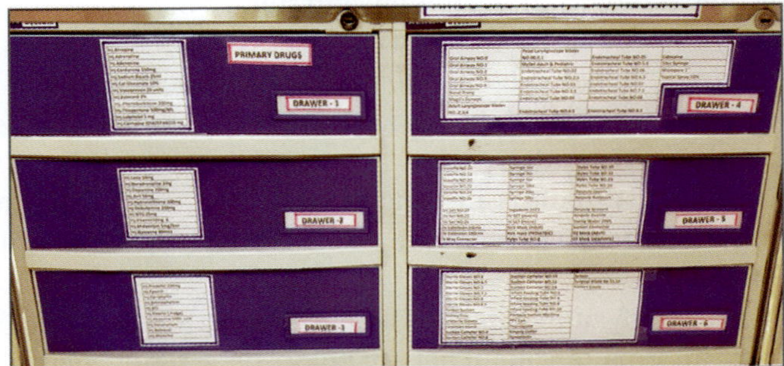

Fig. 1: Emergency medications labeled and stored in crash cart.

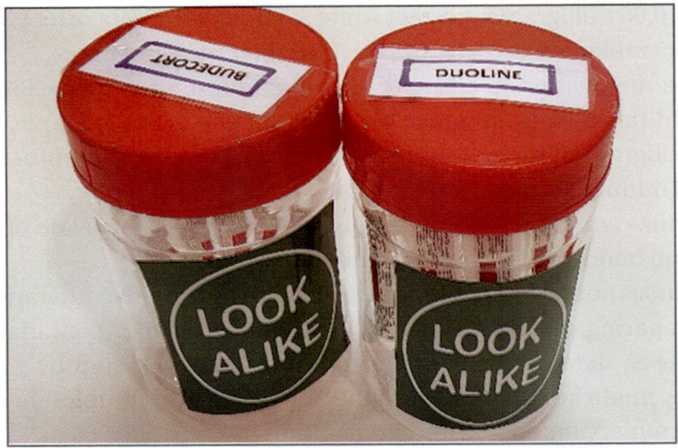

Fig. 2: Look-alike medicines should be labeled properly and stored separately.

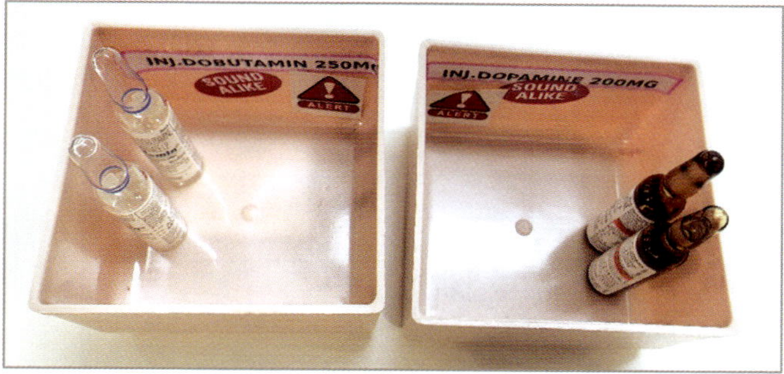

Fig. 3: Soundalike medicines properly labeled and stored separately occupying the opposite corners, and not to be placed closer together.

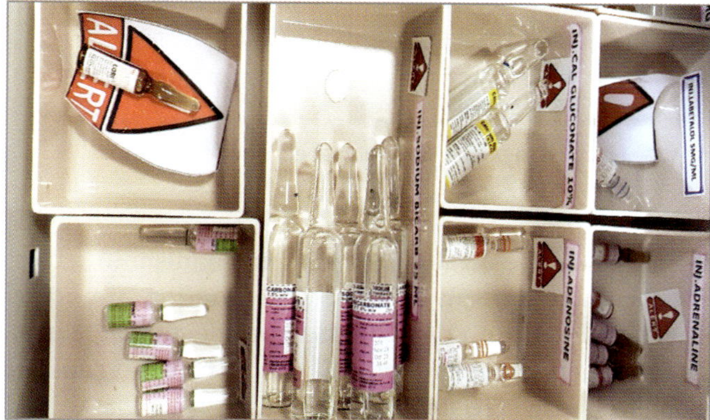

Fig. 4: Additional warning labels to alert staff for drugs with serious side effects.

- Educate staff and patients about look-alikes and soundalikes so that they can watch for errors at outpatient and retail pharmacies. Oral rehydration solution powder is available as 4.4 g sachet and 22 g sachet. The 4.4 g must be dissolved in 200 mL while the 22 g sachet is to be dissolved in 1 L of water. Errors in preparation can lead to serious electrolyte imbalance.

Prevention of drug administration errors:
- To avoid errors in drug administration nurses should be trained to follow the six rights of medication administration: right medication is administered to the right individual, in the right dose, at the right time, via the right route, with the right documentation.
- Nurses also must pay attention to the right reason for the drug to be administered, the date of expiry, and how to store reconstituted medications.
- When intravenous fluids are prepared or two or mode solutions are mixed, a label should be attached to the fluid container with details on the added electrolyte, date, and time of preparation, etc. **(Fig. 5)**.

INFUSION LABEL　　　　　　　Hospital

Name of the Patient ________________________

MPI No. ________________________________

Dept: ____________________ Bed No. ___________

Diluent _________________________________

Additives-Name of the drug ________________

Dosage _________________________________

Calculated Dose/ml _______________________

Total Hours of infusion ___________________

Date and time of preparation ______________

Start Time______________ End Time____________

________________　　　　________________
Prepared by　　　　　　　　Verified by
(Sign and emp ID)　　　　(Sign and emp ID)

Fig. 5: Use of user-friendly labels on preparations.

- Double-checks can be a valuable safety mechanism in reducing errors by checking that the drug dose and preparation are correct before administration. For the double-checks to be effective, at least two people must perform them independently. Checking together runs the risk that both people will make the same error.
- Encourage a NICU culture of identification and reporting of medication errors by staff. Encourage using critical incident reporting forms that are analyzed in a non-punitive manner by a multidisciplinary team.

Use of additional resources for error minimization:
- *Smart infusion pumps*: Smart infusion pumps with software can be programmed to administer a variety of medications and linked to computerized physician order entry.
- A clinical pharmacist adds value to the team by reviewing all medication orders for accuracy (adherence to the neonatal unit formulary), checking for allergy or comorbidities that require dose adjustment and helping nurses with formulations.

Drug Compatibility Chart

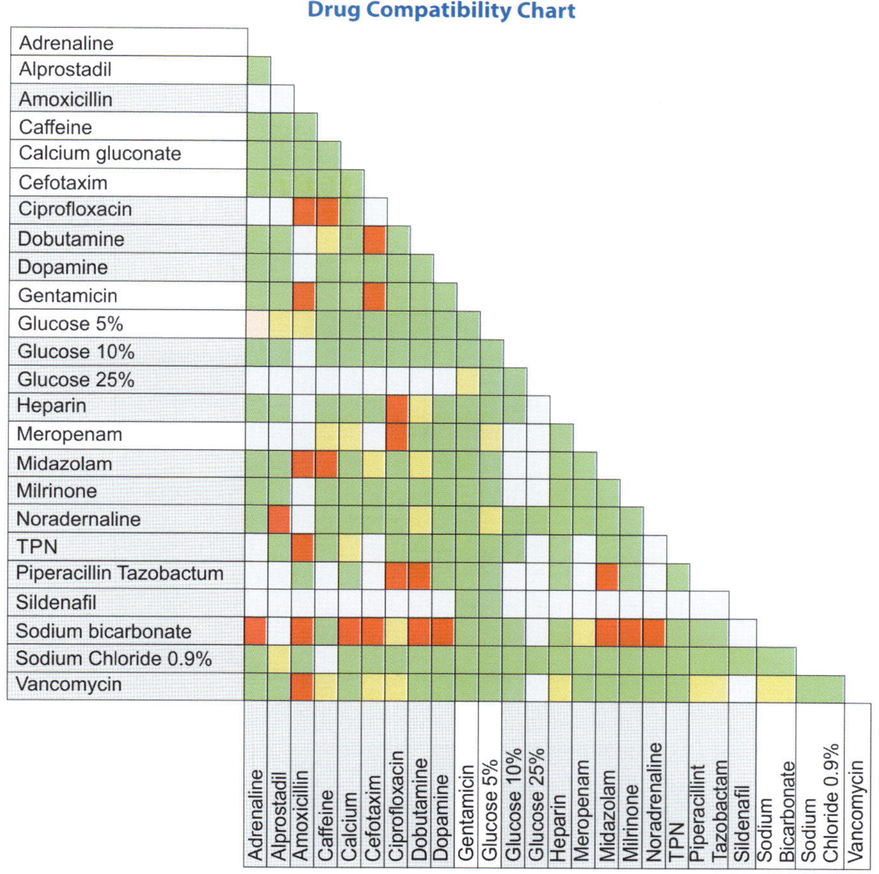

Procedures

▶ Central Lines in Neonate

▶ Peripherally Inserted Central Catheter

▶ Central Line Associated Bloodstream Infections (CLABSI) Prevention Checklist

▶ Chest Tube Insertion

▶ Use of Nebulizer

▶ Kangaroo Mother Care

▶ Retinopathy of Prematurity Screening

Hand Hygiene

■ OBJECTIVE

The participants should be able to perform hand hygiene using appropriate steps in an efficient manner to maintain asepsis in neonatal care.

■ SUPPLIES

- Hand rub
- Running water
- Elbow-operated tap
- Soap
- Posters on steps of hand hygiene and moments of hand hygiene
- Wall clock with seconds watch or a timer

■ STEPS

- Roll up sleeves of the gown/shirt approximately one inch above the elbow.
- Remove all ornaments, bandages, and wristbands.
- Wet hands and forearm by keeping hands below running water/take handful of hand rub.
- Gently rub all the hand surfaces.
- First step is palm to palm.
- Second step is right palm over left dorsum with interlaced fingers and vice versa.
- Third step is palm to palm with fingers interlaced.
- Fourth step is backs of fingers to opposing palms with fingers interlocked.
- Fifth step is rotational rubbing of left thumb clasped in right palm and vice versa.
- Sixth step is rotational rubbing, backward and forward clasped fingers of right hand in left palm and vice versa.
- Wash hands using running water in case of washing with soap and water.
- Allow the hands to air dry.
- If using an elbow-operated tap, close the tap using the elbow.

■ DO'S ✔

- Do give enough time for each step of hand hygiene.
- Do wash your hands with soap and water if hands are visibly soiled and also before doing any sterile procedure.
- Allow the hands to dry before touching the neonate.

■ DON'TS ✖

- Do not touch the neonate with wet hands.
- Do not come back from elbows to hand with the water dripping down as it may touch the non-washed area near elbows.

How to Handrub?

Rub hands for hand hygiene wash hands when visibly soiled

Duration of the entire procedure: 20–30 seconds

1a 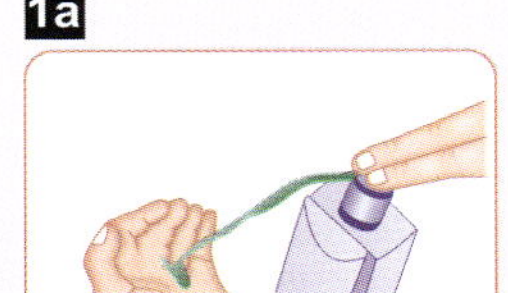

1b 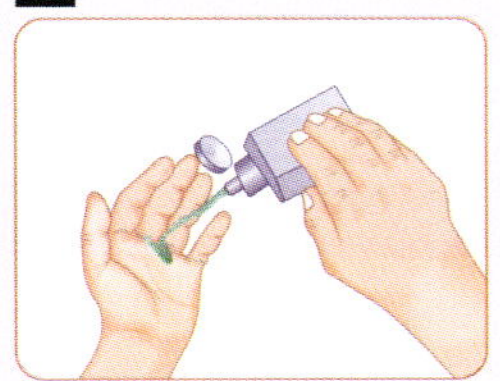

Apply a palmful of the product in a cupped hand, covering all surfaces

2 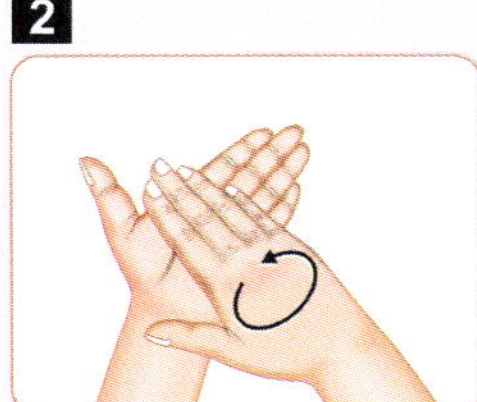

Rub hands palm to palm

3 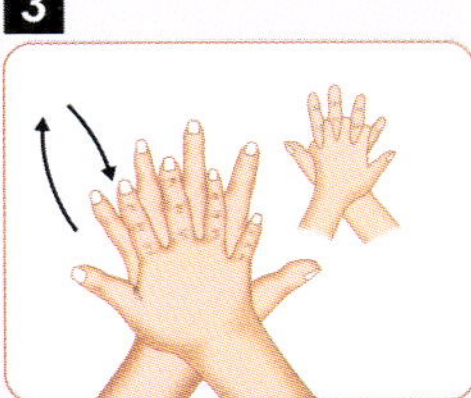

Right palm over left dorsum with interlaced fingers and vice versa

4 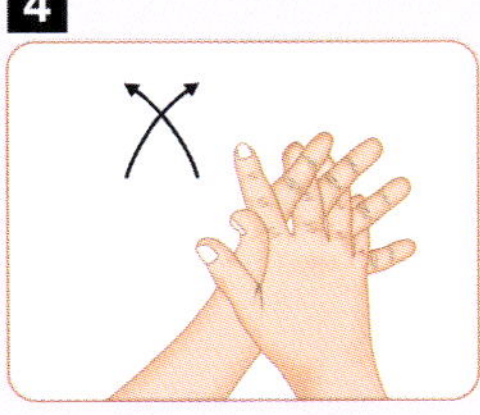

Palm to palm with fingers interlaced

5 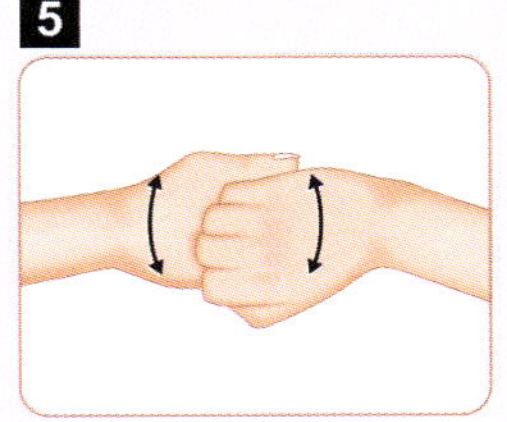

Backs of fingers to opposing palms with fingers interlocked

6 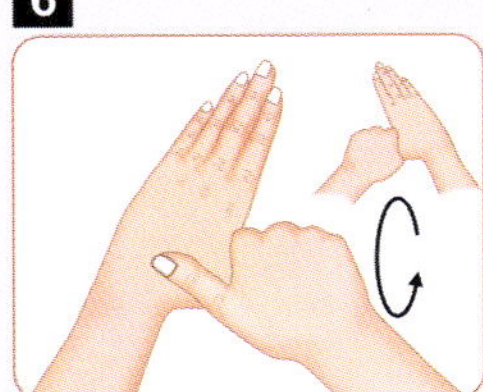

Rotational rubbing of left thumb clasped in right palm and vice versa

7 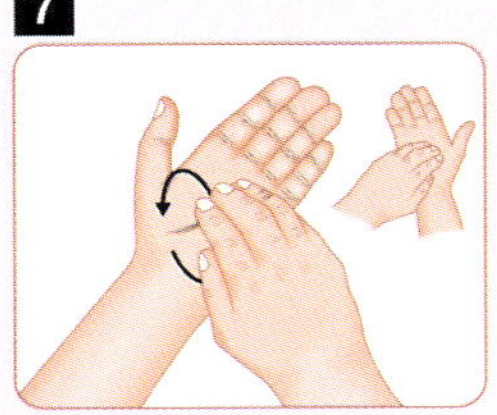

Rotational rubbing, backwards and forwards with clasped fingers of right hand in left palm and vice versa

8 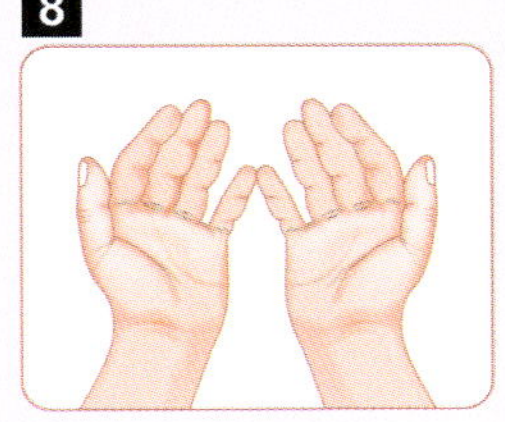

Once dry, your hands are safe

How to Handwash?

Wash hands when visibly soiled! Otherwise, use handrub

Duration of the entire procedure: 40–60 seconds

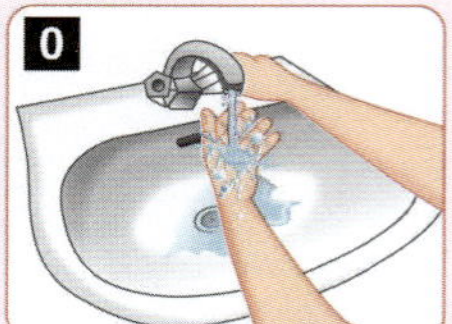

Wet hands with water

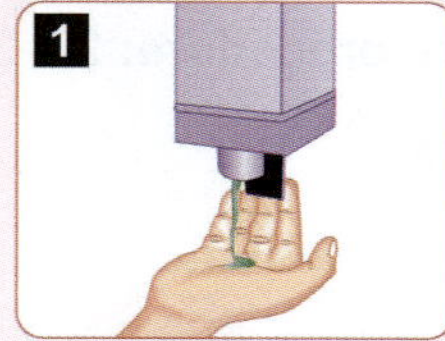

Apply enough soap
to cover all hands surfaces

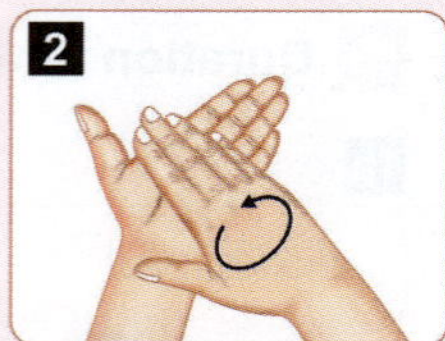

Rub hands
palm to palm

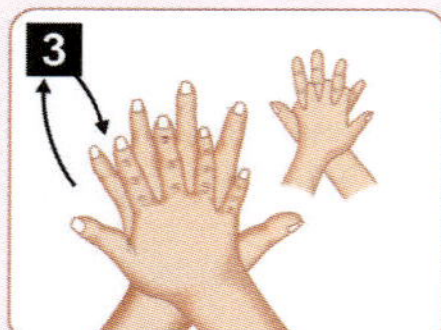

Right palm over left
dorsum with interlaced
fingers and vice versa

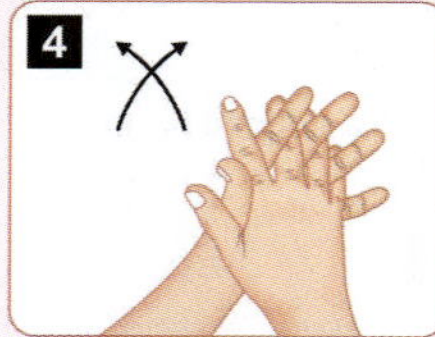

Palm to palm with
fingers
interlaced

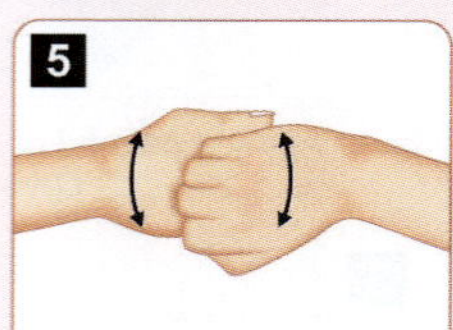

Backs of fingers to
opposing palms with
fingers interlocked

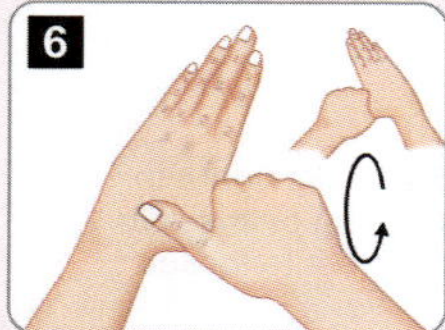

Rotational rubbing of
left thumb clasped in
right palm and
vice versa

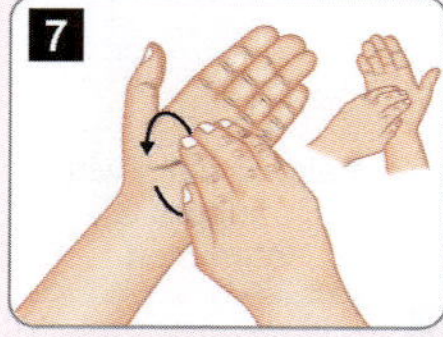

Rotational rubbing,
backwards and forwards
with clasped fingers of right
hand in left palm and vice versa

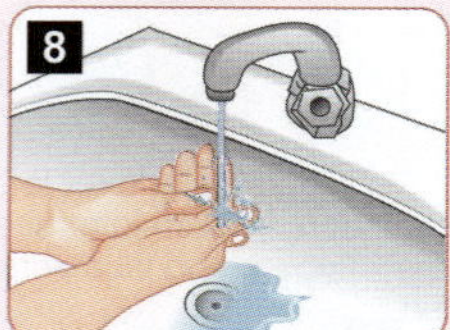

Rinse hands
with water

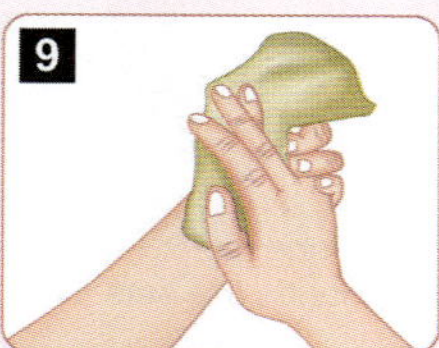

Dry hands thoroughly
with a single use towel

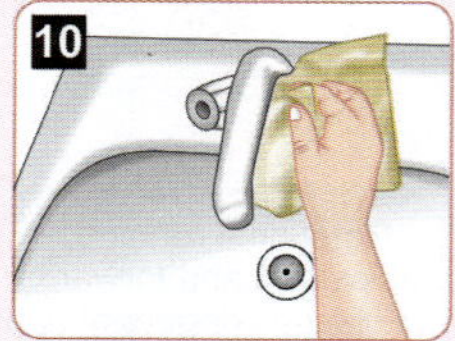

Use towel to turn
off faucet

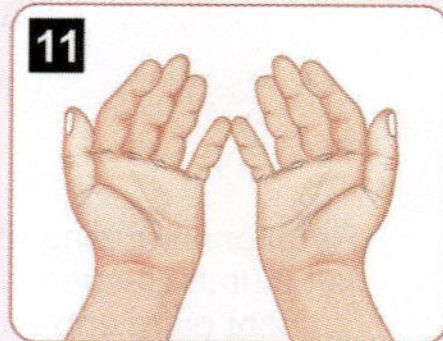

Your hands are
now safe

Your 5 Moments
for Hand Hygiene

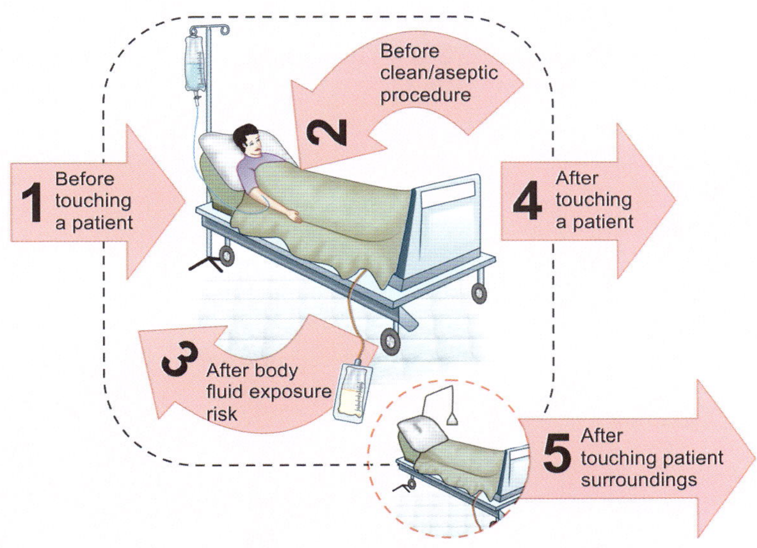

1 **Before touching a patient**	**WHEN?**	Clean your hands before touching a patient when approaching him/her.	
	WHY?	To protect the patient against harmful germs carried on your hands.	
2 **Before clean/aseptic procedure**	**WHEN?**	Clean your hands immediately before performing a clean/aseptic procedure.	
	WHY?	To protect the patient against harmful germs, including the patient's own, from entering his/her body.	
3 **After body fluid exposure risk**	**WHEN?**	Clean your hands immediately after an exposure risk to body fluids (and after glove removal).	
	WHY?	To protect yourself and the healthcare environment from harmful patient germs.	
4 **After touching a patient**	**WHEN?**	Clean your hands after touching a patient and her/his immediate surroundings, when leaving the patient's side.	
	WHY?	To protect yourself and the healthcare environment from harmful patient germs.	
5 **After touching patient surroundings**	**WHEN?**	Clean your hands after touching any object or furniture in the patient's immediate surroundings, when leaving-even if the patient has not been touched.	
	WHY?	To protect yourself and the healthcare environment from harmful patient germs.	

TABLE 1: Objective structured clinical examination (OSCE) for steps of hand hygiene.

S. No	Step	Points (1 each)
1.	Rolls up sleeves of the gown/shirt approximately one inch above the elbow	
2.	Removes all ornaments, bandages, and wristbands	
3.	Wets hands and forearm by keeping hands below running water/take handful of hand rub	
4.	Gently rubs all the hand surfaces	
5.	First step is palm to palm	
6.	Second step is right palm over left dorsum with interlaced fingers and vice versa	
7.	Third step is palm to palm with fingers interlaced	
8.	Fourth step is backs of fingers to opposing palms with fingers interlocked	
9.	Fifth step is rotational rubbing of left thumb clasped in right palm and vice versa	
10.	Sixth step is rotational rubbing, backward, and forward clasped fingers of right hand in left palm and vice versa	
11.	Washes hands using running water in case of washing with soap and water	
12.	Allows the hands to air dry	
13.	If using an elbow-operated tap, closes the tap using the elbow	
	Total (13)	

Performing Venepuncture and Blood Sample Collection

■ OBJECTIVE

The participants should be able to perform venipuncture and collect blood sample from neonates, safe, clean, and efficiently.

■ SUPPLIES

- Two pairs of sterile disposable gloves
- Disposable 5-mL syringe with needle (at least two)
- Swabs or cotton balls soaked in antiseptic solution
- Prelabelled blood collection tubes (vacutainers)
- Lab forms and specimen labels
- Manikin/or venipuncture arm for venipuncture

Asepsis and developmentally supportive care should be a prerequisite for every procedure.

■ STEPS (FIG. 1)

- Gather the supplies.
- Ensure adequate lighting.
- Wash hands and put on sterile gloves.
- The cover of the gloves may be used as a sterile base on which the swabs, needle etc., can be placed.

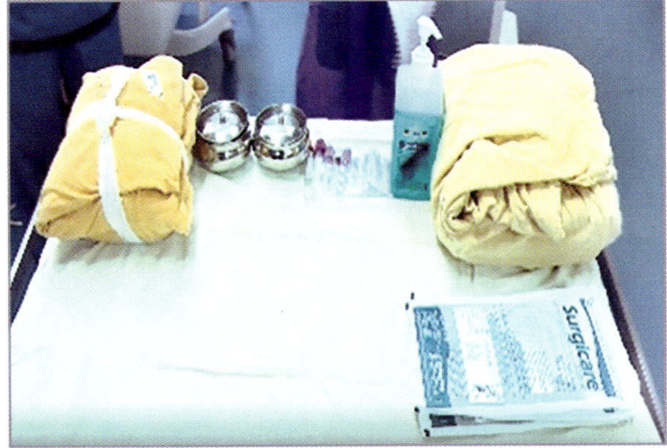

Fig. 1: Gather the supplies.

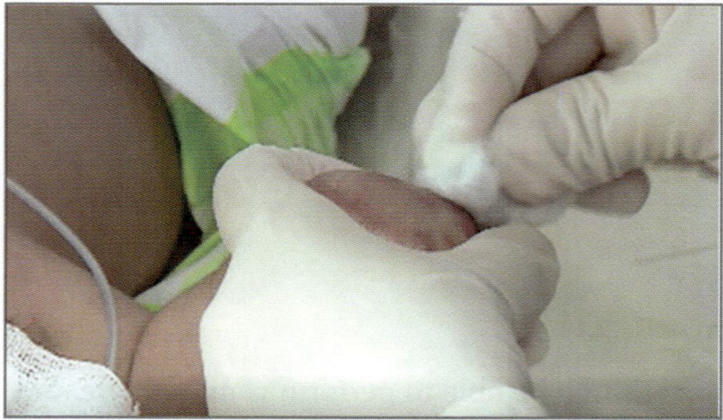

Fig. 2: Skin preparation before venepuncture.

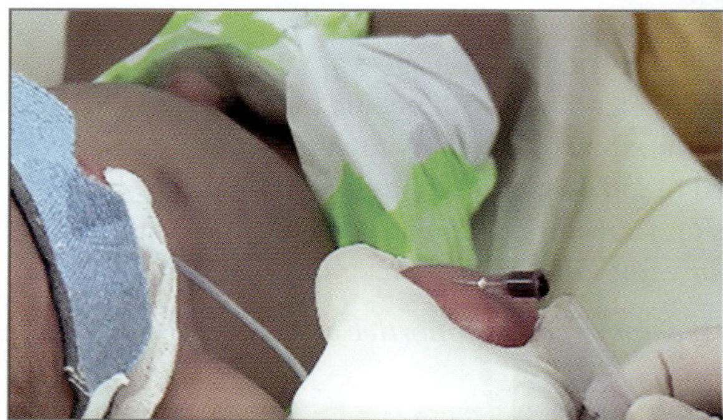

Fig. 3: Hold the needle so that it slowly fills the needle with blood.

- Identify a suitable vein, the more periphery the better.
- Sterilize the area—use a single swab or triple swab method (Povidone-Iodine/Chlorhexidine)/prepare the insertion site with >0.5% chlorhexidine in an alcohol solution, using a back-and-forth motion for a minimum of 30 seconds, and allow to dry completely **(Fig. 2)**.
- Allow it to dry for 30 seconds.
- Stretch the skin and hold it firmly with nondominant hand.
- Insert needle (Gauge 23 or 24) 3–5 mm distal to (away from) the vein and advance till you observe flashback of blood.
- If the needle enters alongside the vein rather than into it, withdraw the needle slightly without removing it completely, and angle it into the vessel.
- Pull back very slightly on syringe and hold so that it fills slowly to collect the amount needed with 5-mL syringe attached to needle **(Fig. 3)**.
- Press the site with dry cotton for few seconds to avoid oozing of blood at venipuncture site **(Fig. 4)**.
- Fill the tube with the sample and label it.
- Discard the waste in biomedical waste bins as per protocols **(Fig. 5)**.
- Wash hands and document the procedure.

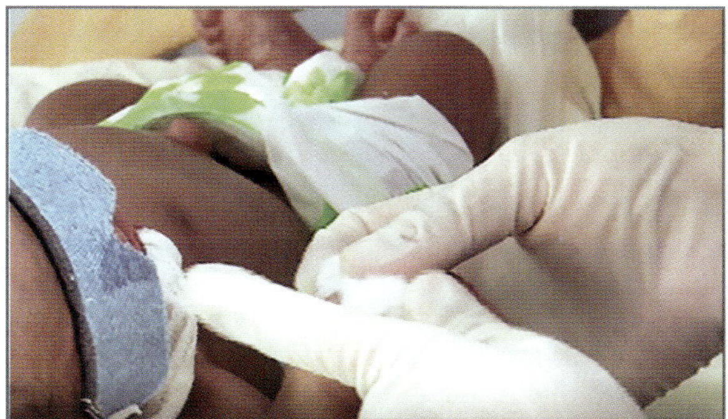

Fig. 4: Press the site with dry cotton and hold.

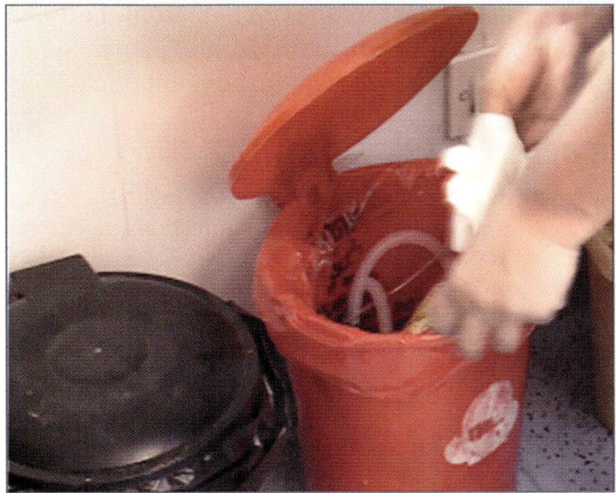

Fig. 5: Discard the waste as per biomedical waste management.

■ DO'S ✓

- Follow the non-pharmacological pain relief measures and developmentally supportive care **(Fig. 6)**.
- Fresh disposable needle should be used for taking the culture sample.

■ DON'TS ✕

- Palpate the area of puncture after the site preparation.
- Needle of the syringe used for drawing sample should not touch the hub of needle.

■ MONITORING AND CARE

- Assess the puncture site for ongoing bleeding.

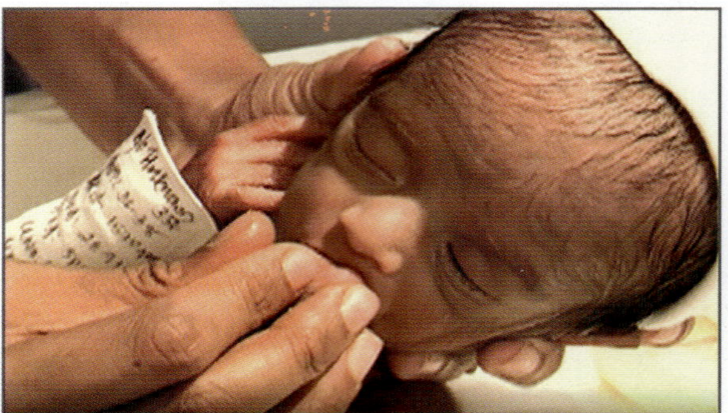

Fig. 6: Follow the non pharmacological pain measures.

- Assess previously used puncture sites for hematoma and signs of infection (e.g., redness, swelling, warmth, drainage, and pain at the puncture site).
- Assess perfusion in the extremity where the venepuncture was performed.

■ FURTHER READING/VIEWING

1. Lai NM, Lai NA, O'Riordan E, Chaiyakunapruk N, Taylor JE, Tan K. Skin antisepsis for reducing central venous catheter-related infections. Cochrane Database Syst Rev. 2016;7:CD010140.
2. Shah D, Tracy M. Skin antisepsis survey in Australia–New Zealand neonatal nurseries. J Paediatr Child Health. 2013; 49:601-2.
3. Tamma PD, Aucott SW, Milstone AM. Chlorhexidine use in the neonatal intensive care unit: results from a national survey. Infect Control Hosp Epidemiol. 2010;31:84.
4. YouTube. Available from https://m.youtube.com/watch?v=Lmzkg04FX4Q [Last accessed March, 2024].

TABLE 1: Objective structured clinical examination (OSCE) for venipuncture.

S. No.	Steps	Points (1 each)
1.	Gathers the supplies	
2.	Washes hands and puts on sterile gloves	
3.	Forms a sterile base using the cover of gloves, and places the supplies needed on it	
4.	Identifies a suitable peripheral vein	
5.	Sterilizes the area—use a single swab or triple swab method	
6.	Allows it to dry for 30 seconds	
7.	Stretches the skin and hold it firmly with nondominant hand	
8.	Inserts needle and observe flashback of blood	
9.	Collects the amount of blood needed using the needle and the syringe without touching the hub of the inserted needle	
10.	Presses the site with dry cotton for few seconds to avoid oozing of blood	
11.	Empties the syringe blood into the tube and labels it	
12.	Discards the waste in respective biomedical waste bins as per protocols	
13.	Discards the sharp needle into plastic container (sharp pit)	
14.	Washes hands and documents the procedure	
	Total (14)	

Peripheral Intravenous Vein Catheterization

■ OBJECTIVE

The participants should practice the insertion of IV line for sample collection, intravenous fluid administration, medications, and blood transfusion.

■ SUPPLIES

- Two pairs of sterile gloves **(Fig. 1)**
- Sterile intravenous catheter of 24–26G **(Fig. 2)**
- Sterile infusion set with intravenous fluid **(Fig. 3)**.

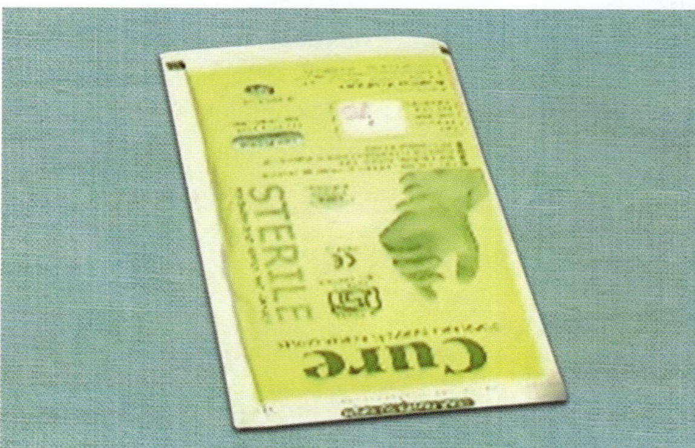

Fig. 1: Pair of sterile gloves.

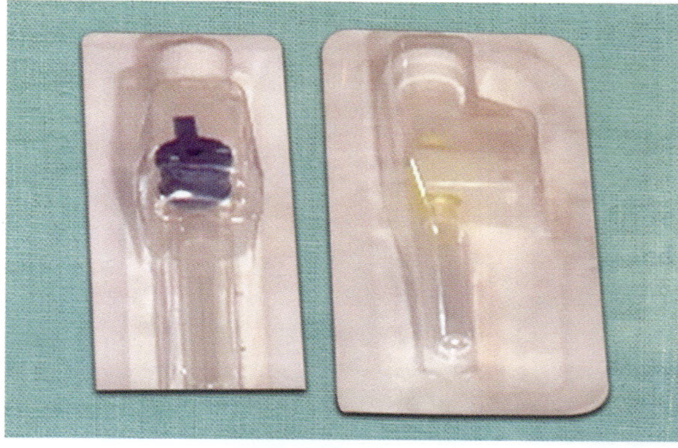

Fig. 2: Sterile intravenous catheter.

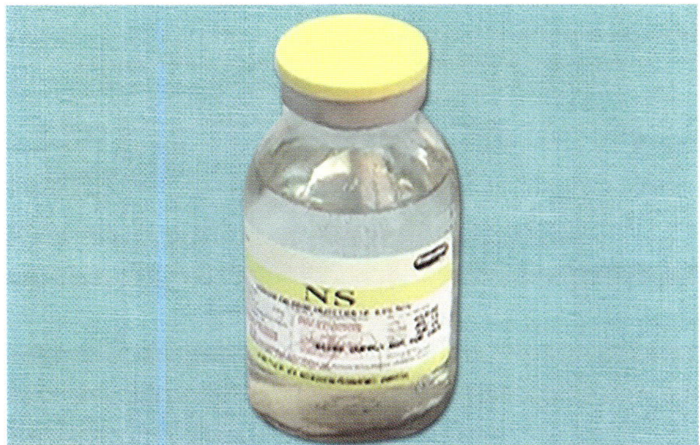

Fig. 3: Infusion set with intravenous fluid.

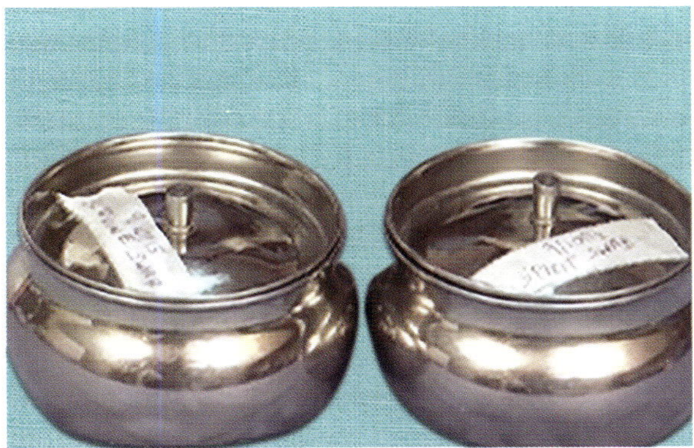

Fig. 4: Swabs or cotton balls soaked in antiseptic solution

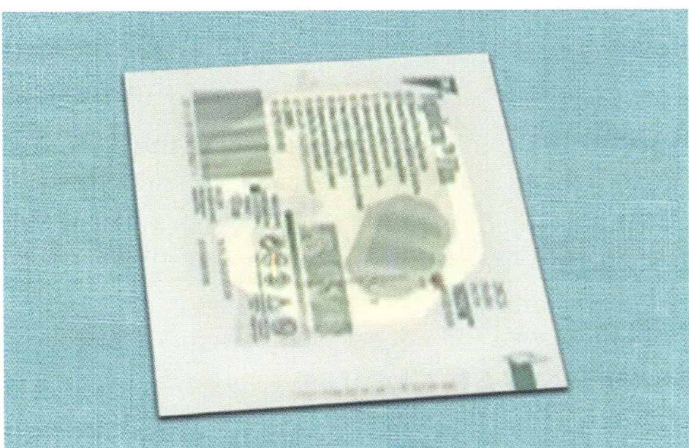

Fig. 5: Adhesive tape.

- Sterile 1, 2, 5, and 10-mL syringe (at least two each)
- Swabs or cotton wool balls soaked in antiseptic solution **(Fig. 4)**.
- Adhesive tape **(Fig. 5)**
- Syringe with normal saline.

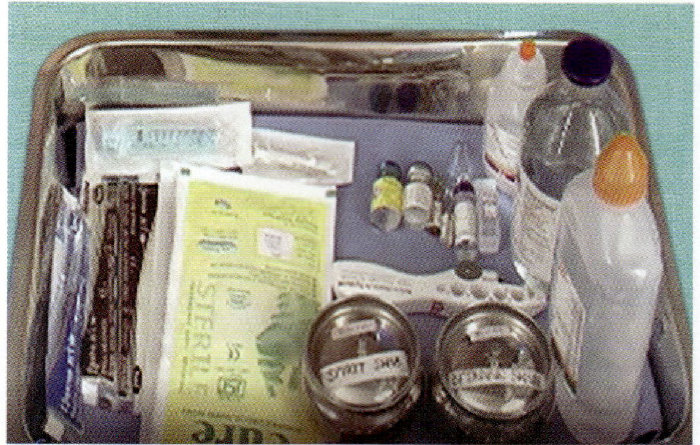

Fig. 6: Collect all the supplies needed, in a sterile tray.

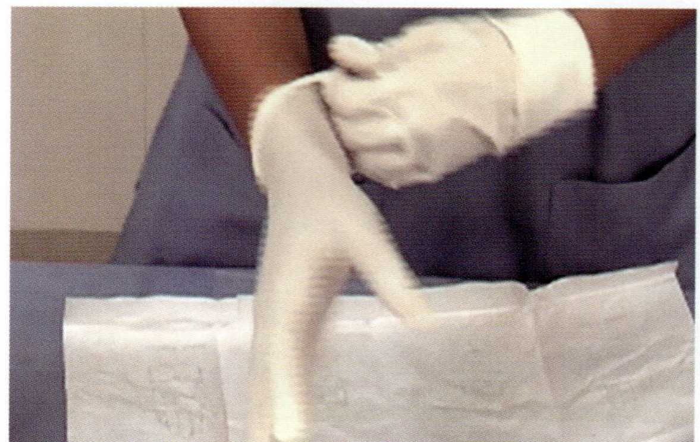

Fig. 6: Collect all the supplies needed, in a sterile tray.

■ STEPS

- Identify an accessible vein, most commonly on the dorsum of hand, foot, or antecubital area.
- Collect all the items needed for peripheral vein catheterization **(Fig. 6)**.
- Perform hand hygiene and wear gloves **(Fig. 7)**.
- Create a sterile area at the bedside/tray.

■ WEAR STERILE/CLEAN GLOVES

- Assistant helps in peeling off outer a sterile covers of the disposables.
- Prepare the identified area with single swab applying for 30 seconds or three swabs technique using spirit swab.
- Allow it to dry.
- Insert peripheral intravenous vein catheterization (PIVC) by picking tip of PIVC at an angle to skin surface **(Figs. 8 and 9)**.
- After the PIVC is inserted completely, withdraw the needle **(Fig. 10)**.

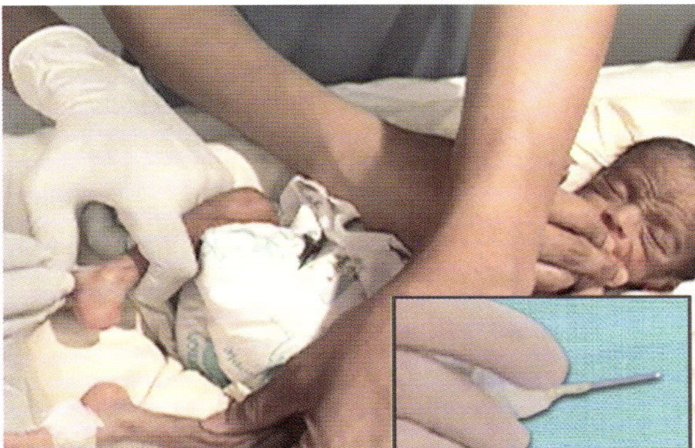

Fig. 8: Insert the iv cannula holding it an angle towards the skin.

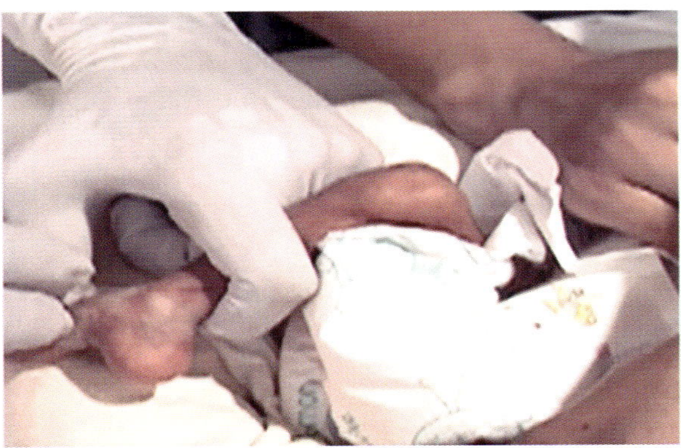

Fig. 9: Insert the iv cannula at an angle.

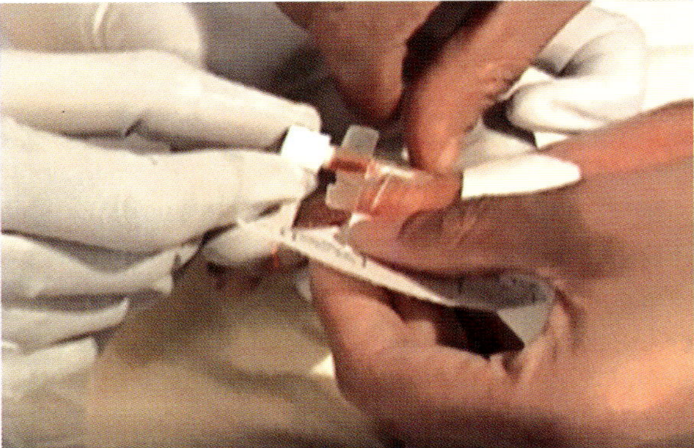

Fig. 10: Withdraw the needle after inserting cannula.

- Flush the PIVC with 0.5–1 mL of normal saline **(Fig. 11)**.
- Fix the PIVC with semi-transparent adhesive.
- Fix the rear end of PIVC with usual dressing such as Durapore or micropore.

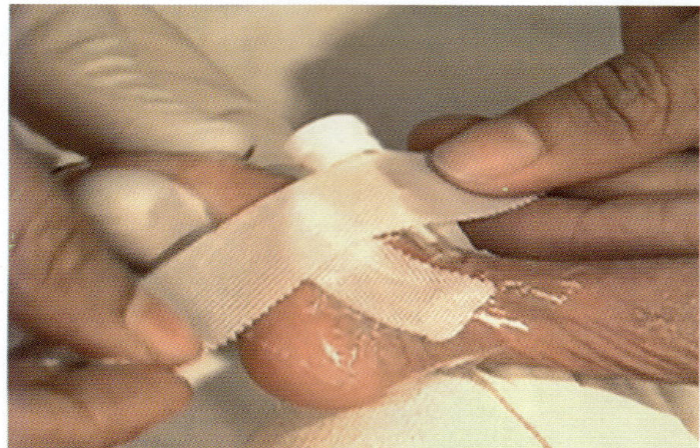

Fig. 11: Fix the PIVC using a semi transparent tape.

- Can use splint only when its cannula is placed at a mobile joint area.
- Put the date of insertion of PIVC on the adhesive.
- Discard the waste in biomedical waste bin as per protocol.
- Wash hands and document the procedure.

■ DO'S ✅

- Make sure that the key part of the disposable (tip of IV cannula) does not come in contact with non-sterile area.
- Follow nonpharmacological measures for pain relief.
- Keep the overlying skin clean and dry.
- Monitor in each shift and before any administration, for redness or tenderness of surrounding skin.

■ DON'TS ❌

- Do not touch the prepared area and if touched, perform the cleaning steps again.

■ FURTHER READING

1. CDC. 2017. Recommendations | BSI | Guidelines Library | Infection Control, 2017. Available from: https://www.cdc.gov/infectioncontrol/guidelines/bsi/recommendations.html [Last accessed March, 2024].
2. Lai NM, Lai NA, O'Riordan E, Chaiyakunapruk N, Taylor JE, Tan K. Skin antisepsis for reducing central venous catheter-related infections. Cochrane Database Syst Rev. 2016;7:CD010140.
3. NICU, CDC. 2020. NICU: S. aureus Guidelines | Infection Control |, 2020. Available from: https://www.cdc.gov/infectioncontrol/guidelines/nicu-saureus/index.html [Last accessed March, 2024].
4. YouTube. Available from: https://www.youtube.com/watch?v=C10YBMvg7Ew [Last accessed March, 2024].

S. No.	Steps	Points (1 each)
	TABLE 1: Objective structured clinical examination (OSCE) for peripheral intravenous vein catheterization (PIVC).	
1.	Identifies an accessible vein	
2.	Collects all the items needed for peripheral vein catheterization	
3.	Performs hand hygiene	
4.	Creates a sterile area at the bedside/tray	
5.	Wears sterile/clean gloves	
6.	Makes sure none of the parts of disposables (key parts) come in contact with non-sterile area	
7.	Prepares the identified area with single swab applying for 30 seconds or three swabs technique using spirit swabs	
8.	Allows it to dry	
9.	Inserts PIVC by picking tip of PIVC at approximately 30–45° angle to skin surface	
10.	After the PIVC is inserted completely, withdraw the needle	
11.	Flushes the PIVC with 0.5–1 mL of normal saline	
12.	Fixes the PIVC with semi-transparent adhesive	
13.	Fixes the rear end of PIVC with usual dressing such as Durapore or micropore	
14.	Puts the date of insertion of PIVC on the adhesive	
15.	Discards the waste in biomedical waste bin as per protocol	
16.	Washes hands and documents the procedure	
	Total (16)	

Dextrose Monitoring

OBJECTIVE

The participants should be able to monitor dextrose in a neonate in a safe and efficient manner.

SUPPLIES

- Two pairs of sterile gloves **(Fig. 1)**
- Spirit swabs **(Fig. 2)**
- Lancets/needles (24G)
- Glucometer with dextrostix

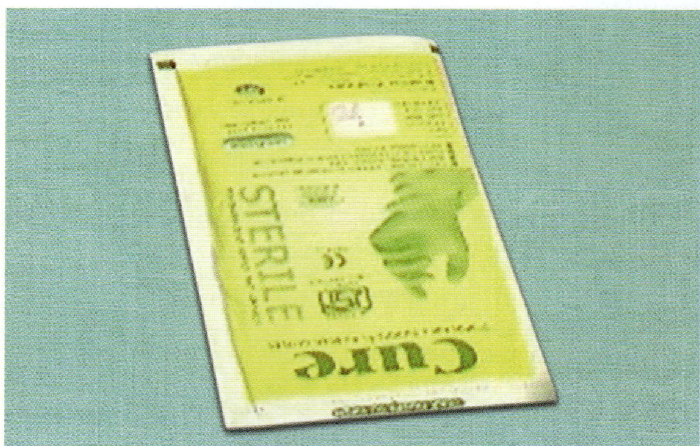

Fig. 1: Sterile gloves.

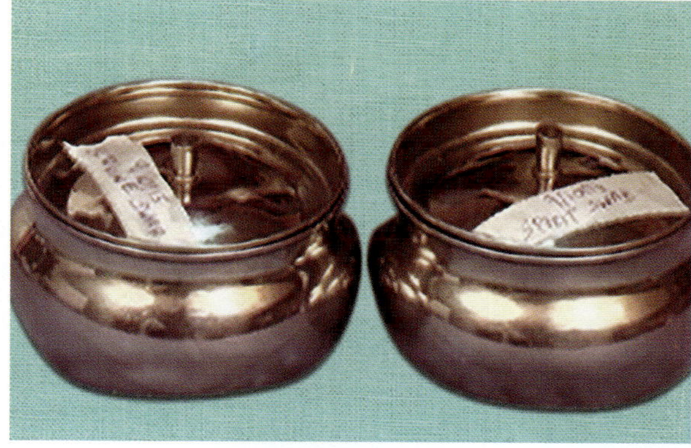

Fig. 2: Spirit and povidone iodine swabs.

STEPS

- Consider applying eutectic mixture of local anesthetic (EMLA) cream 45 minutes before the procedure or consider giving expressed breast milk during the procedure, KMC, nonnutritive sucking for analgesia.
- Perform hand hygiene using alcohol-based hand rubs.
- Ask for helper, the helper opens sterile procedure tray on a clean surface/trolley.
- Arrange spirit or chlorhexidine swabs.
- Helper strip opens a 24G disposable hypodermic needle and hands it over to the bedside nurse.
- Nurse places the needle inside the tray using aseptic non-touch-technique.
- Helper gives Glucostrip to the bedside nurse in similar manner. Helper places the glucometer-glucose strip assembly close to the tray taking care that glucose strips do not touch anywhere to protect the key part.
- Nurse holds glucose strip, and the helper holds glucometer and the two negotiate Glucostrip in the glucometer to actuate it.
- Prepare the heel of the neonate by rubbing spirit swab for 30 seconds in a circular fashion starting from the area of interest. After that allow the area to try for 30 seconds.
- Perform heel lancing.
- Allow the drop to build up sufficiently before touching the tip of glucose strip with the blood drop **(Fig. 3)**.
- After the procedure apply a dry cotton ball to press the point of puncture **(Fig. 4)**.
- Discard the biomedical waste in the respective bag.
- Document the procedure in notes.

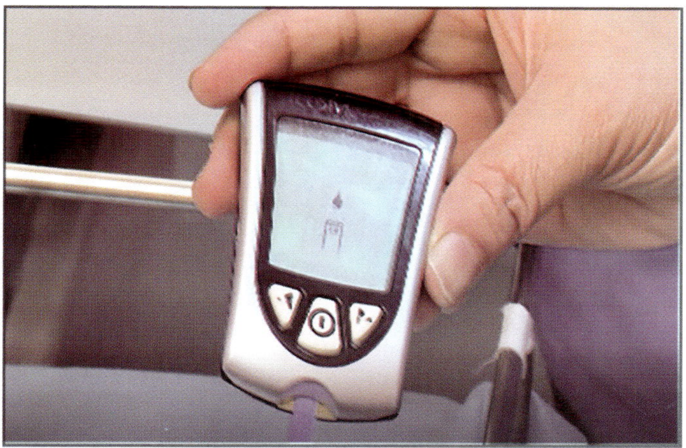

Fig. 3: Wait for the glucometer reading after putting the drop of blood.

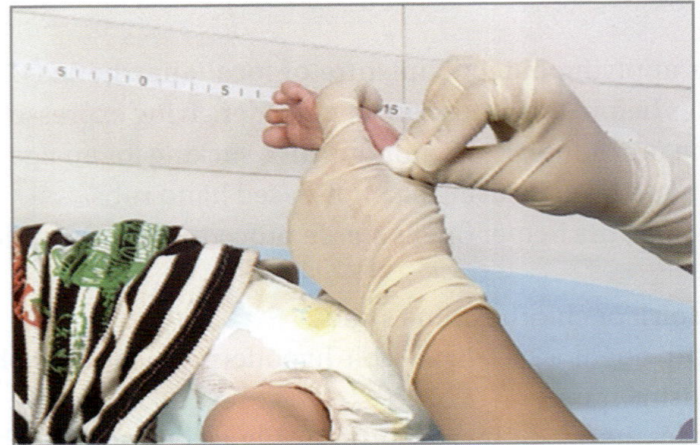

Fig. 4: After the prick, hold the puncture site with dry cotton.

■ DO'S ✔

- Do give enough time for the antiseptic to dry before pricking for dextrose monitoring as excessive antiseptic may interfere with glucose values.
- Prewarming the area will help in free flow of blood to form an adequate droplet for proper dextrose monitoring.

■ DON'TS ✖

- Do not prick at the center of heel as it has vascular anastomosis and damage can cause calcaneal necrosis.
- Do not squeeze hard to withdraw the blood.

TABLE 1: Objective structured clinical examination (OSCE) for dextrose monitoring.

S. No.	Steps	Points (1 each)
1.	Considers applying eutectic mixture of local anesthetic (EMLA) cream 45 minutes before the procedure or considers giving expressed breast milk during the procedure, KMC, non-nutritive sucking for analgesia	
2.	Performs hand hygiene using alcohol-based hand rubs	
3.	Asks for helper, the helper opens sterile procedure tray on a clean surface/trolley	
4.	Arranges spirit or chlorhexidine swabs	
5.	Helper strip opens a 24G disposable hypodermic needle and hands it over to the bedside nurse	
6.	Nurse places the needle inside the tray using aseptic non-touch-technique	
7.	Helper gives Glucostrip to the bedside nurse in similar manner. Helper places the glucometer-glucose strip assembly close to the tray taking care that glucose strips does not touch anywhere to protect the key part	
8.	Nurse holds glucose strip, and the helper holds glucometer and the two negotiate Glucostrip in the glucometer to actuate it	
9.	Prepares the heel of the neonate by rubbing spirit swab for 30 seconds in a circular fashion starting from the area of interest. After that allow the area to try for 30 seconds	
10.	Performs heel lancing	
11.	Allows the drop to build up sufficiently before touching the tip of glucose strip with the blood drop	
12.	After the procedure applies a dry cotton ball to press the point of puncture	
13.	Discards the biomedical waste in the respective bag	
14.	Documents the procedure in notes	
	Total (14)	

Blood Culture

■ OBJECTIVE

The participants should be able to perform venepuncture and collect blood sample for blood culture from neonates safely and efficiently.

■ SUPPLIES (FIG. 1)

- Two pairs of sterile disposable gloves
- Disposable 24G and 26G needle
- Disposable 2-mL and 5-mL syringe with needle
- Swabs or cotton balls soaked in antiseptic solution
- Pre-labelled blood culture bottles
- Laboratory forms and specimen labels
- Manikin/or venepuncture arm for venepuncture.

■ STEPS

- Identify an accessible vein, most commonly on dorsum of hand or foot or antecubital vein **(Fig. 2)**.
- Collect all the items needed for blood culture.
- Perform hand hygiene.
- Create a sterile area at the bedside/tray.
- Wear sterile/clean gloves.

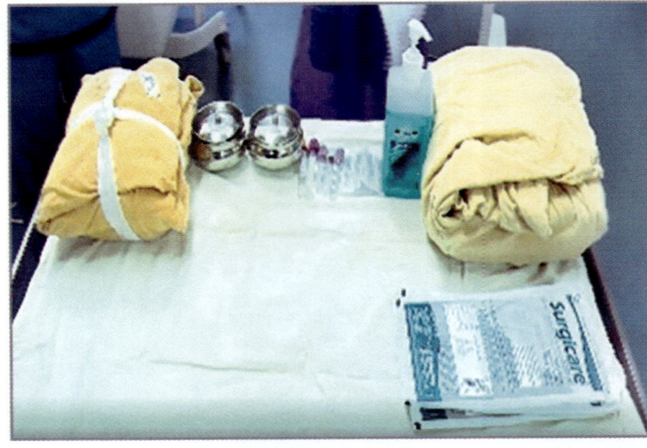

Fig. 1: Gather all supplies.

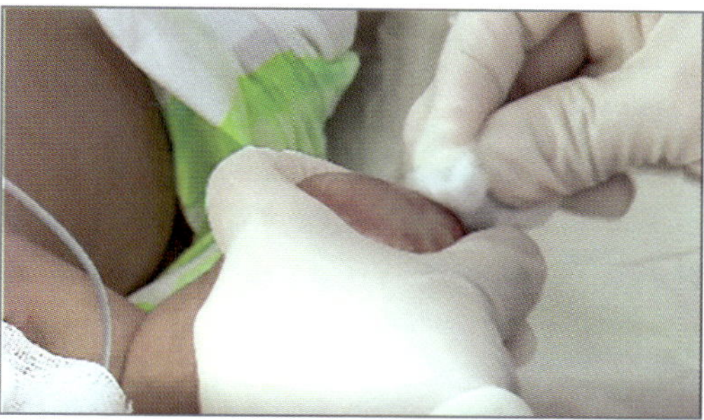

Fig. 2: Identify an accessible vein.

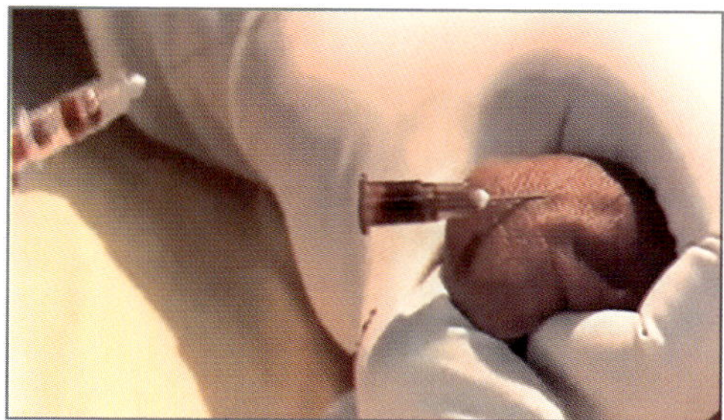

Fig. 3: Once needle fills with blood, withdraw using a syringe.

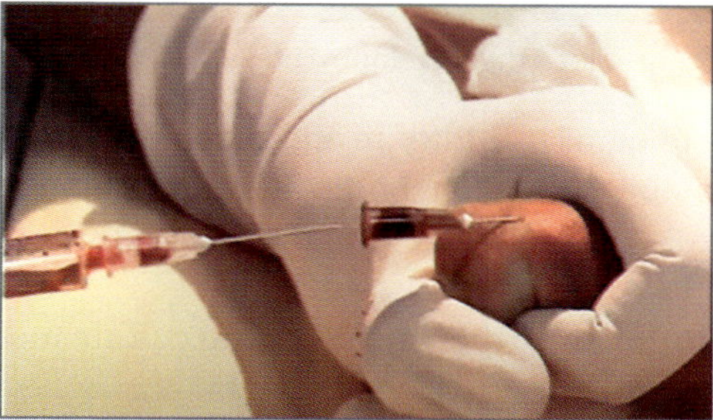

Fig. 4: Once needle fills with blood, withdraw using a syringe.

- Prepare a circular area of skin approximately 5 cm diameter over the proposed puncture site by cleaning the area (three spirit swabs or chlorhexidine swabs).
- Allow it to dry.
- Indicate that cleaning would be in concentric circles moving outwards from the center.
- Puncture the vein with 24G or 26G needle.
- Do not break the hub of the needle.
- Once blood starts flowing freely, gently withdraw the blood using a 2-mL syringe and needle **(Figs. 3 and 4)**.
- Place the needle of the 2-mL syringe inside the hub of first needle and withdraw the drop of blood.
- Withdraw about 1–2 mL of blood.

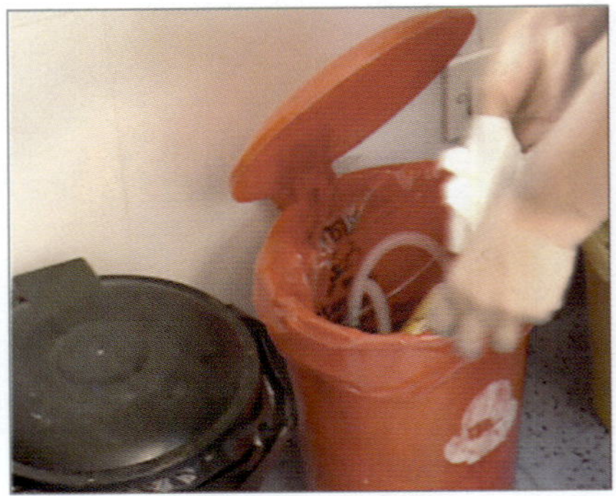

Fig. 5: Discard the waste in appropriate bag.

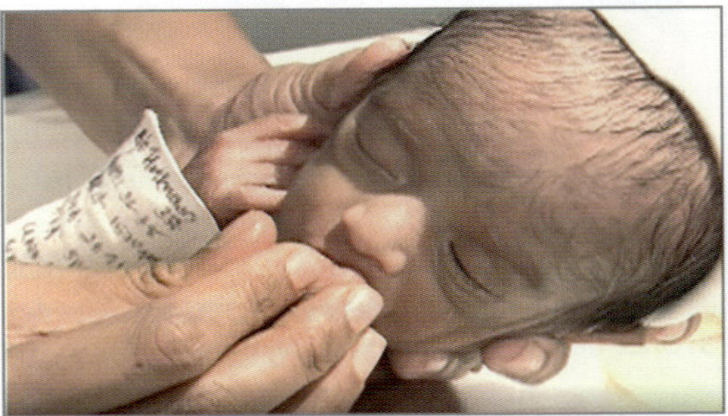

Fig. 6: Follow the developmentally supportive care.

- Check for absence of turbidity in the blood culture bottle media and indicate that blood to be put in bottle only if no turbidity.
- Insert the needle of the syringe into the cap and slowly inject the blood into bottle.
- Shake the bottle gently to mix the blood and culture media.
- Label the samples.
- Ensure transfer to the lab immediately (maximum in next 12–24 hours).
- Remove gloves.
- Document the procedure the patient file with date and time.
- Discard the waste in the appropriate waste bag **(Fig. 5)**.

■ DO'S ✔

- Follow the nonpharmacological pain relief measures and developmentally supportive care **(Fig. 6)**.
- Fresh disposable needle should be used for taking the culture sample.

■ DON'TS ✖

- Palpate the area of puncture after the site preparation.
- Needle of the syringe used for drawing sample should not touch the hub of needle.

SpO$_2$ Monitoring

■ OBJECTIVE

The participants should be able to measure oxygen saturation using pulse oximetry in a neonate safely and efficiently.

■ INDICATIONS

- Any neonate receiving oxygen therapy
- Any sick neonate admitted in neonatal care unit
- During resuscitation of a neonate
- During transport of a neonate within the facility or to another facility

■ SUPPLIES

- Hand rub for hand hygiene
- Pulse oximeter **(Fig. 1)**
- Neonatal pulse oximeter probe

■ STEPS

- Perform hand hygiene.
- Identify the indications for using pulse oximeter.
- Go to the setting menu of pulse oximeter and choose the alarm settings **(Fig. 2)**.
- Dial the upper alarm to 95 and lower to 90.
- Ensure that the alarm volume is on and not muted.

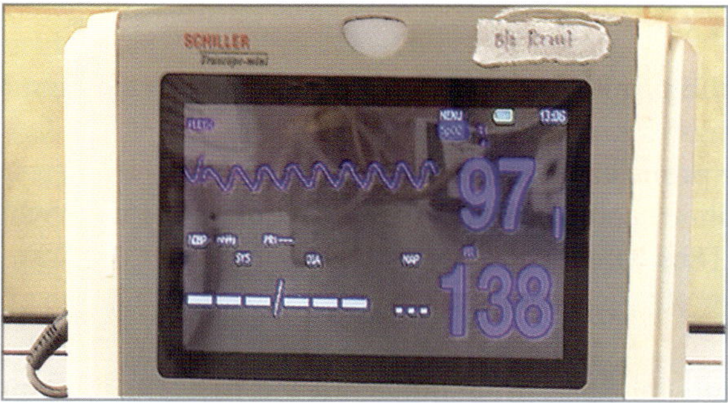

Fig. 1: Pulse oximeter.

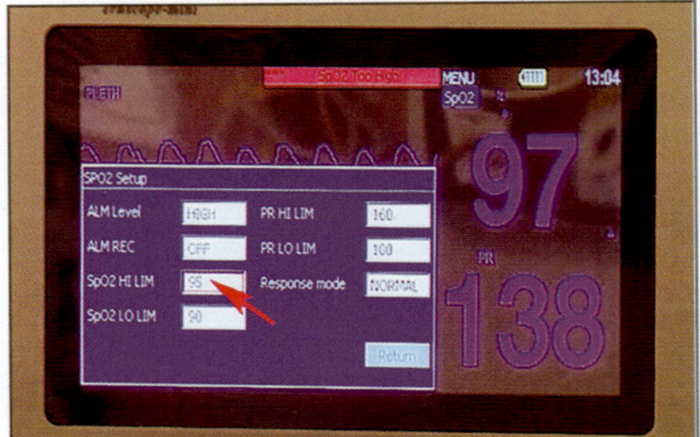

Fig. 2: Setting the alarms.

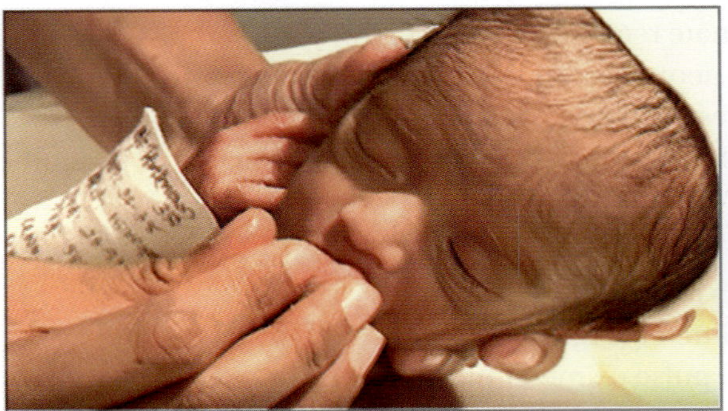

Fig. 3: Nonpharmacological measures to calm the neonate.

- Put the probe into the right palm/wrist of the newborn.
- Attach the neonatal probe to the oximeter.
- Plug the pulse oximeter to the power. Turn it on.
- Note the reading.
- Interpret reading and identifies hyperoxia and hypoxia.
- Know the causes of erroneous values with pulse oximeter.

■ DO'S ✓

- Wait for the proper plethysmograph to appear on screen before noting the readings.
- Clean the probe each time before using it.
- Use nonpharmacological measures to calm the neonate while measuring the SpO_2 **(Fig. 3)**.

■ DON'TS ✗

Do not measure the SpO_2 when the neonate is irritable or crying. Wait for the neonate to calm down.

TABLE 1: Objective structured clinical examination (OSCE) for SpO$_2$ monitoring.

S. No.	Steps	Points (1 each)
1.	Performs hand hygiene	
2.	Identifies the indications for using pulse oximeter	
3.	Goes to the setting menu of pulse oximeter and chooses the alarm settings	
4.	Dials the upper alarm to 95 and lower to 90	
5.	Ensures that the alarm volume is on and not muted	
6.	Puts the probe into right pam/wrist of the newborn	
7.	Attaches the neonatal probe to the oximeter	
8.	Plugs the pulse oximeter to the power. Turn it on	
9.	Notes the reading	
10.	Interprets reading and identifies hyperoxia and hypoxia	
11.	Knows the causes of erroneous values with pulse oximeter	
	Total (11)	

Noninvasive Blood Pressure Monitoring

■ OBJECTIVE

The participants should be able to measure blood pressure (BP) using noninvasive method in neonates safely and efficiently.

■ SUPPLIES

- Hand rub for hand hygiene
- Appropriate size cuff
- Multipara monitor with option for non-invasive BP measurement.

■ STEPS

- Perform hand hygiene.
- Measure the length of right upper arm from the acromion process of scapula to humeral condyle.
- Choose the smallest cuff size that covered at least two-thirds of the right upper arm length and encompassing the entire arm circumference.
- Apply appropriately sized cuff to the right upper arm with baby.
- Ensure that neonate is calm.
- Connect the appropriate noninvasive blood pressure (NIBP) connector to the monitor and press "measure" BP button.
- Record three successive BP recordings at 2-minute intervals.
- Calculate the average of these three readings, rounded off to the nearest mm Hg.
- Document the value in the case sheet.

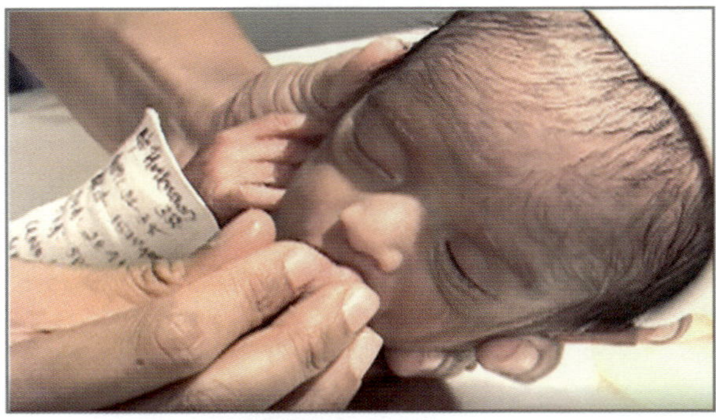

Fig. 1: Nonpharmacological measures for developmentally supportive care.

DO'S 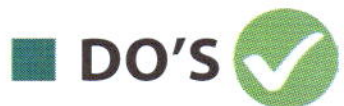

- Follow the non-pharmacological pain relief measures and developmentally supportive care **(Fig. 1)**.

DON'TS

- Do not measure the BP when the neonate is irritable or crying. Wait for the neonate to calm down.

TABLE 1: Objective structured clinical examination (OSCE) for noninvasive blood pressure monitoring.

S. No.	Steps	Points (1 each)
1.	Performs hand hygiene	
2.	Measures the length of right upper arm from acromion process of scapula to humeral condyle	
3.	Chooses the smallest cuff size that covered at least two-thirds of the right upper arm length and encompassing the entire arm circumference	
4.	Applies appropriately sized cuff to the right upper arm with baby in prone position	
5.	Ensures that neonate is calm	
6.	Connects the appropriate NIBP connector to the monitor and press "measure" BP button	
7.	Records three successive BP recordings at 2-minute intervals	
8.	Calculates the average of these three readings, rounded off to the nearest mm Hg	
9.	Documents the value in the case sheet	
	Total (9)	

Orogastric Tube Insertion

■ OBJECTIVE

The participants should be able to insert orogastric tube in neonates safely and efficiently.

■ SUPPLIES

- Hand rub for hand hygiene
- Pair of sterile gloves
- Appropriate size orogastric feeding tube (FG 8 for >2,000 g weight neonates and 5–6 FG for neonates <2,000 g)
- 10-mL/20-mL syringe
- Measuring tape
- Measured amount of feed to be given to be kept ready.
- Stethoscope

■ STEPS

- Perform hand hygiene.
- Select the appropriate size orogastric tube.
- Position the baby supine with head elevated.
- Measure the length of tube to be inserted from the bridge of the nose to the tip of ear lobe and from the ear lobe to a point midway between the xiphoid process and the umbilicus **(Fig. 1)**.
- Mark the tube with measuring or maintain the mark with thumb and finger.

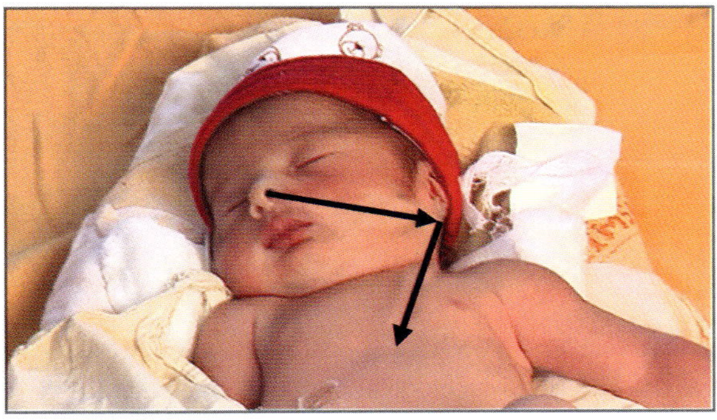

Fig. 1: Measurement of orogastric tube insertion.

- Insert the tube into the mouth until it reaches the premeasured mark on the tubes; uses EBM or baby's saliva as lubricant.
- Check the position of the tube by gently aspirating the stomach contents or by inserting 0.5–1.0 mL of air into stomach while auscultating.
- Bring the tube at the corner and fixes the tube in "C" shape manner **(Fig. 2)**.
- Measure the amount of feed to be given.
- Remove the plunger of the syringe and connect the barrel to the gastric tube.
- Fill the barrel of the syringe with the required amount of milk.
- Allow the milk to run down the tube by gravity.
- Observe the baby during the entire gastric feed, stops the feed if the infant vomits, becomes floppy or developed breathing difficulty.
- Cap the end of tube after feeding. Can open the tube after 30 minutes if on CPAP.
- Discard the waste in appropriate color-coded bag.
- Document on nurses' chart.

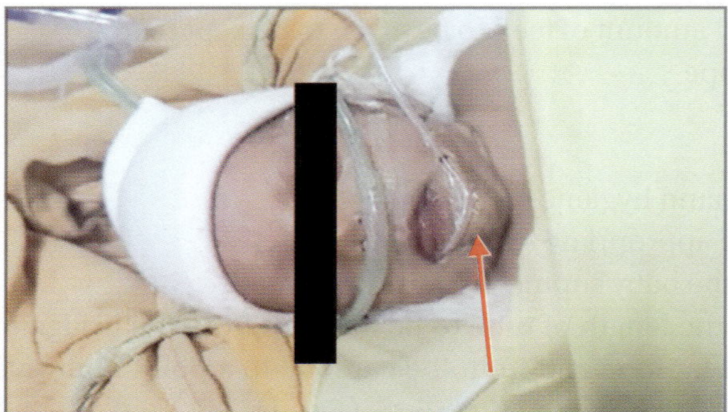

Fig. 2: C type fixation.

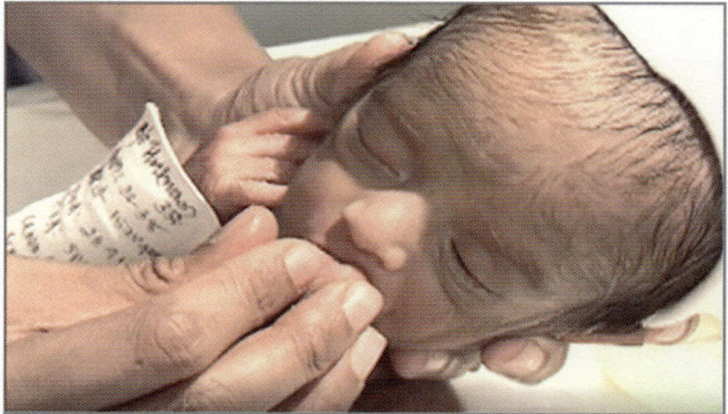

Fig. 3: Use non pharmacological measures of pain management.

■ DO'S ✓

- Wait for the feed to flow with gravity.
- Use nonpharmacological measures to keep the neonate calm while feeding **(Fig. 3)**.

■ DON'TS ✗

- Do not force the feeds by pushing the plunger.

■ FURTHER READING

1. Deorari AK. Practical Procedures for the Newborn Nursery A Manual for Physicians and Nurses AIIMS - NICU Protocols. 4th edition. Noble Vision; 2017.
2. YouTube. Preterm care package, good nutrition. Available from: https://youtu.be/ZDXXDi4Xyjw [Last accessed March, 2024].

TABLE 1: Objective structured clinical examination (OSCE) for orogastric tube insertion.

S. No.	Steps	Points (1 each)
1.	Performs hand hygiene	
2.	Selects the appropriate size orogastric tube	
3.	Positions the baby supine with head elevated	
4.	Measures the length of tube to be inserted from the bridge of the nose to the tip of ear lobe and from the ear lobe to a point midway between the xiphoid process and the umbilicus	
5.	Marks the tube with measuring or maintains the mark with thumb and finger	
6.	Inserts the tube into the mouth until it reaches the premeasured mark on the tubes; uses EBM or baby's saliva as lubricant	
7.	Checks the position of the tube by gently aspirating the stomach contents or by inserting 0.5–1.0 mL of air into stomach while auscultating	
8.	Brings the tube at the corner and fixes the tube in "C" shape manner	
9.	Measures the amount of feed to be given	
10.	Removes the plunger of the syringe and connects the barrel to the gastric tube	
11.	Fills the barrel of the syringe with required amount of milk	
12.	Allows the milk to run down the tube by gravity	
13.	Observes the baby during the entire gastric feed, stops the feed if the infant vomits, becomes floppy or developed breathing difficulty	
14.	Caps the end of tube after feeding. Can open the tube after 30 minutes if on CPAP	
15.	Discards the waste in appropriate color coded bag	
16.	Documents on nurses' chart	
	Total (16)	

Lumbar Puncture

■ OBJECTIVE

The participants should be able to perform lumbar puncture (LP) and collect cerebral spinal fluid (CSF) safely and efficiently in all indicated neonates.

■ SUPPLIES

- Surgical gloves—two pairs
- Surgical gowns/cap/mask
- Sterile drapes/disposable sheets—three
  - One with the hole to increase the visibility for LP site
- Sterile containers—four in number
- LP needle/sterile disposable 23G/24G/26G needle
- Laboratory forms and specimen labels
- Anti-septic solution
- Sterile sponges for preparing the site
- Mannequin for lumbar puncture

■ INDICATIONS

- Suspected central nervous system (CNS) infections (bacterial, fungal, and viral)
- Neonatal seizures/encephalopathies (nonketotic hyperglycemia)
- Hydrocephalous (to relieve intracranial pressure in rapidly growing variety)
- Administration of intrathecal medications

■ CONTRAINDICATIONS

- Hemodynamic/cardiovascular instability
- Severe respiratory distress
- Soft tissue infection at the site of LP
- Bleeding diathesis
- Lumbosacral deformities
- Increased intracranial pressure

■ STEPS

Procedure

- *Analgesic:* Use sterile gauge soaked in 24% sucrose/25% glucose or breast milk. Other topical agents can be applied 30 minutes before the procedure.
- *Position:* Keep the neonate in lateral recumbent position as shown in **Figure 1**.
  - Place the child on their side near the edge of bassinet in lateral decubitus position.
  - Draw the knees upward and flex by placing one arm of the assistant over the knees and back of the baby. Stabilize the neck and flex by placing the other arm of assistant over the neck. Ensure that the neck is not hyperflexed.
  - Spine should be visualized and avoid undue rotation. Avoid too much pressure until the needle is about to be inserted.
- *Aseptic precautions:*
  - Personnel doing the procedure should wear a cap, mask and follow proper hand hygiene and then wear sterile gown.
  - Both personnel should wear the sterile gloves.
  - Clean the area (including the iliac crests area) with appropriate solution as per the hospital policy. Allow it to dry.
  - Apply the drapes to maintain asepsis as shown in **Figure 2**.
  - Make a hole in the disposable sheet if it is not having.
- *Identify the site:*
  - First identify the posterior-superior iliac crests (PSIC) (arrow mark represents in **Figure 3**).
  - Draw an imaginary line between the posterior superior iliac crests. The line corresponds to L4 in neonates (red dotted line represents).
- Sterile needle has to be inserted in the midline slightly toward head at angle of 70–90° through L3/L4 or L4/L5 intervertebral space aiming toward the umbilicus with a steady pressure and non-rotatory movement **(Fig. 4)**.

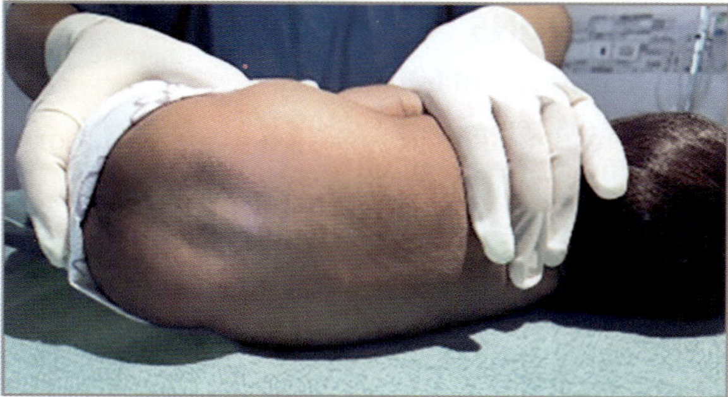

Fig. 1: Lateral recumbent position.

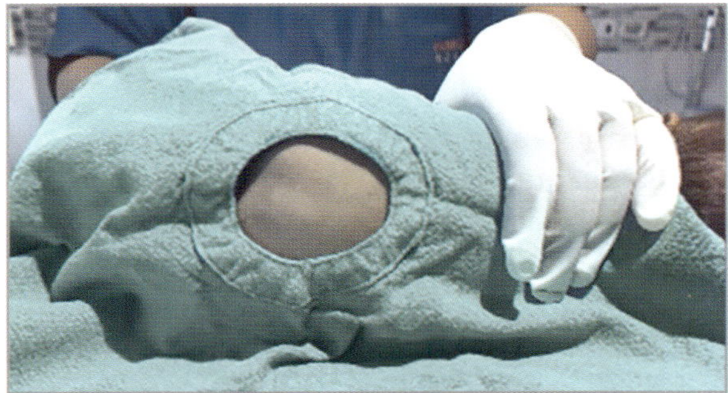

Fig. 2: Position and aseptic precautions for lumbar puncture.

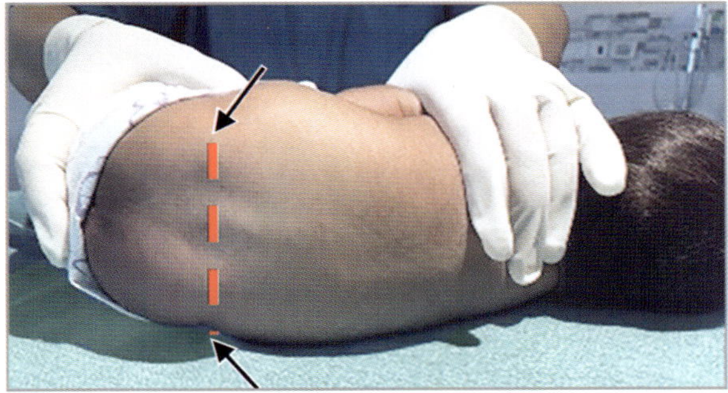

Fig. 3: Showing posterior-superior iliac crests (PSIC) and L4.

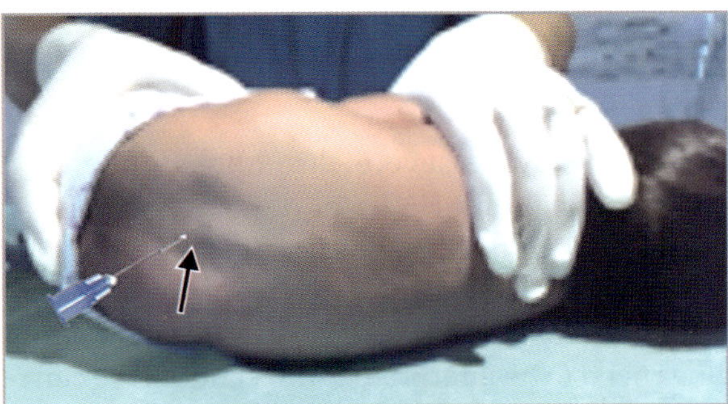

Fig. 4: Needle placement and direction.

- After entering the skin, allow the neonate to settle, reorient and move forward.
- Advance the needle by 0.5–1.0 cm till you see CSF coming.
- Collect CSF in sterile container. A minimum of 10 drops/tube is required for microbiological and biochemical sterile containers and about 1–1.5 mL for culture.
- For a therapeutic tap, we can remove volume up to 2% of body weight (3–5 mL/kg body weight).

- Remove the needle slowly after you got adequate sampling.
- Apply the pressure on the site to prevent ooze.
- Reposition the neonate gently.
- After the ooze ceases, apply sterile dressing.
- Monitor the vitals of the neonate.
- Discard the biomedical waste generated in the procedure properly.
- Wash hands and document the procedure.

If a bloody specimen is obtained:
- If the CSF becomes clearer in subsequent container, then is most likely a traumatic LP. Adjustment of WBC counts in a traumatic LP does not aid in the diagnosis of meningitis in neonates.
- If blood does not clear in subsequent container and clot is formed, then most likely a vein is punctured. Repeat in a different space.
- If blood does not clear and no clot is formed, then it is due to intracranial bleed.
  Repeat the LP after 24–48 hours.

■ DO'S ✅

- Monitor the neonate throughout the procedure.
- Abandon the procedure if neonate had developed apnea and desaturation.
- A disposable needle can be used for doing LP when special needles are not available.
- Take the consent from parents/guardian prior to procedure.

■ DON'TS ❌

- Avoid in children having severe thrombocytopenia (<20,000) and deranged coagulation profile (INR >1.5)
- Do not draw the CSF from LP needle after insertion.
- Do not touch the hub of the needle.
- *Traumatic LP with blood in CSF:* Can be used for microbiological culture. Other findings need to be interpreted with caution. We can repeat LP after 24–48 hours if needed.

■ FURTHER READING

1. Deorari AK. Practical Procedures for the Newborn Nursery A Manual for Physicians and Nurses AIIMS - NICU Protocols. 4th edition. Noble Vision; 2017.
2. UpToDate. (2019). Lumbar puncture: Indications, contraindications, technique, and complications in children. Available from: https://www.uptodate.com/contents/lumbar-puncture-indications-contraindications-technique-and-complications-in-children [Last accessed March, 2024].

TABLE 1: Objective structured clinical examination (OSCE) for lumbar puncture.

S. No.	Steps	1 point each
1.	Takes the consent from parents/guardian	
2.	Gathers the supplies	
3.	Washes hands and wear sterile attire properly	
4.	Uses analgesia before starting procedure according to unit protocol	
5.	Asks the assistant to keep the baby in lateral recumbent position	
6.	Sterilizes the area with antiseptic solution. Allows it to dry for 30 seconds	
7.	Identifies posterior-superior iliac crest and identifies L4 vertebra	
8.	Insert a sterile needle slowly towards head in L3/L4 or L4/L5 space	
9.	Stabilizes the neonate and collect CSF into sterile containers.	
10.	Removes the needle slowly	
11.	Applies the pressure over the site and apply dressing after ooze ceases	
12.	Brings the baby back to supine position and document vitals	
13.	Removes the sterile attire and dispose the biomedical waste properly	
14.	Washes the hands and document the procedure	
15.	Writes the laboratory requisition and labels the containers for laboratory	
	Total (15)	

Exchange Transfusion

This SOP is designed to improve the knowledge, skills, and clinical practice of all stakeholders involved in the care of neonates needing blood exchange transfusion.

◼ AIM OF PROCEDURE

To learn about:
- How to prepare for blood exchange transfusion **(Box 1)**.
- How to do blood exchange transfusion **(Box 2)**.

BOX 1: Preparation and equipment.

- Obtain informed consent from parents/guardian
- Obtain blood samples of baby and mother for cross match
- Arrange for the blood as per the chart given below **(Table 1)**
- Umbilical catheter selection as per weight
  3.5 Fr: <1 kg, 4 Fr: 1–2 kg, 5 Fr: 2–3 kg, 7 Fr: >3 kg
- Sterile gloves (two pairs)
- Dressing set
- Cap/mask/gown (two pairs)
- Spirit/betadine/chlorhexidine 2%
- Drapes (2)
- Syringe 2 mL (2), 5 mL (2), 10 mL (2), 20 mL (2)
- IV cannula 24 No. (1)
- Three-way stop cock (2)
- Blood transfusion set
- IV set (2)
- Plastic or glass bottle for disposal of blood
- Saline/sterile water
- Transparent dressing
- Paper tape/Tegaderm/Durapore
- Surgical blade
- Sucrose analgesia?
- Exchange cycle chart prepared
- Cycle volume and cycle number determined
- Pulse oximeter/monitor attached
- Resuscitation equipment checked **(Figs. 1A and B)**

BOX 2: Steps of the procedure.

- Take informed consent from parents
- Insert a peripheral IV line if not already in place
- Blood to be checked for fresh blood (collected within 72 hours), blood group as per requirement
- Blood bag number and blood group cross-checked
- Keep blood at room temperature if blood warmer is not available
- Aspirate stomach contents before the procedure if fed within 4 hours
- The baby's legs and hands are held in position with a cotton drape
- Clean the umbilicus with spirit-betadine-spirit or chlorhexidine swab
- Clean the procedure area and drape with three sterile sheets so that only the umbilical area is visible
- Tie a gauze piece at the base of the umbilicus loosely
- Cut the umbilicus at 1 cm above the base with the clean surgical blade; if the cord has dried up, we may need to cut at the base carefully avoiding the skin
- Identify the umbilical vein is identified at 11 o'clock position
- Cannulate the umbilical vein with a pre-saline-filled umbilical catheter attached to three-way cannula
- Take proper aseptic precautions during cannulation
- Keep umbilical catheter in-situ after ensuring free flow of blood
- Connect the three-way connected to umbilical catheter
- If umbilical catheter insertion is unsuccessful insert peripheral artery cannula
- Ensure blood bag is sufficiently warm
- Connect transfusion set and IV set properly **(Figure 2A to C)**
- Start first cycle with pull out
- Push same volume in
- Mix the bag intermittently
- Monitor the hemodynamic during the procedure
- Do the desired number of cycles
- Ensure blood volume was sufficient for cycles
- Send the last aliquot for PCV, TSB
- Write the procedure notes
- Note any complication during the procedure in the document

TABLE 1: Chart for reference for issue of blood for exchange transfusion.

Baby blood group	Mother's blood group	Blood to be issued
O	O	O
	A	O
	B	O
	AB	O
A	O	O
	A	A, O
	B	O
	AB	A, O

Contd…

Contd...

Baby blood group	Mother's blood group	Blood to be issued
B	O	O
	A	O
	B	B, O
	AB	B, O
AB	O	O
	A	A, O
	B	B, O
	AB	AB, B, A, O
Rh Positive	Rh positive	Rh positive
	Rh negative	Rh negative
	Rh positive	Rh negative
Rh Negative	Rh negative	Rh negative

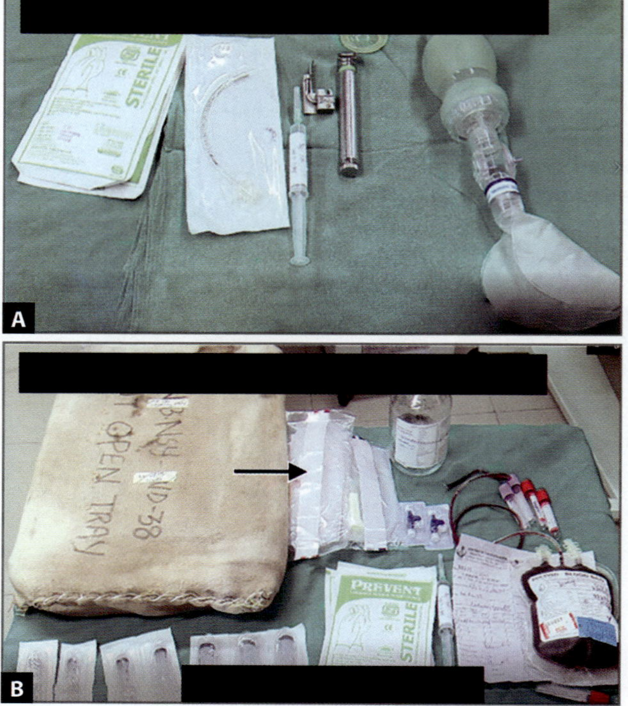

Figs. 1A and B: Keep the resuscitation and suction equipment ready before the procedure.

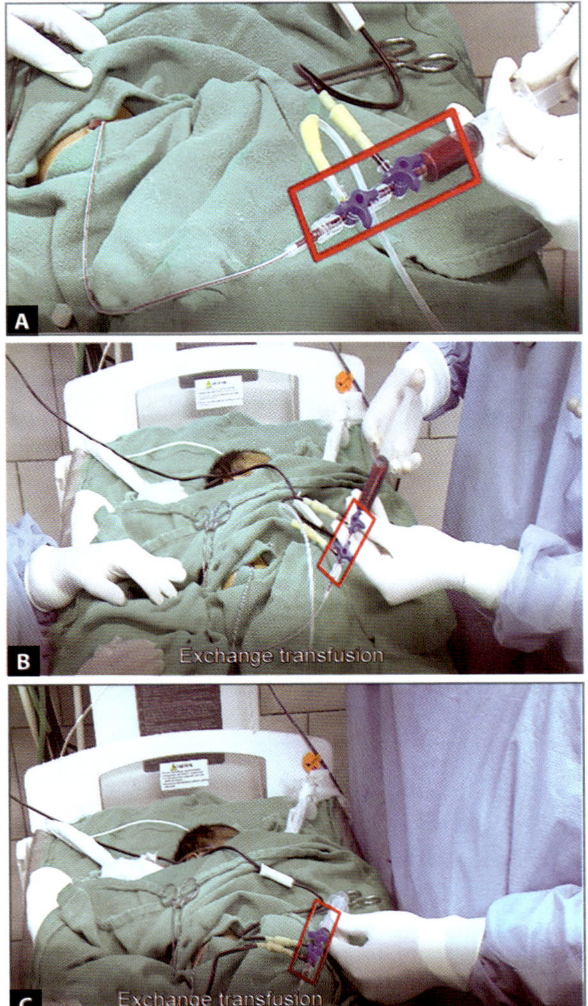

Figs. 2A to C: Position of stop cock (connect proximal stop cock, which is toward the umbilicus to the discarded bottle, connect distal stop cock, which is away from umbilicus to the fresh whole blood). (A) *Step 1:* Pull out baby's blood; (B) *Step 2:* Discard the pulled-out blood; (C) *Step 3:* Pull in fresh blood and push into the baby.

■ FURTHER READING

1. Kapoor D, Singh P, Seth A. Current perspective on exchange transfusion. Indian Pediatr. 2017;54(11):961-2.
2. Murki S, Kumar P. Blood exchange transfusion for infants with severe neonatal hyperbilirubinemia. Semin Perinatol. 2011;35(3):175-84.
3. Newbornwhocc.org. Preterm care package. Available from: https://youtu.be/42xzmYqkjB4 [Last accessed March, 2024].

S. No.	Steps	1 point each
	TABLE 2: Objective structured clinical examination (OSCE) for exchange transfusion.	
1.	Gathers supplies	
2.	Inserts peripheral cannula	
3.	Checks for fresh blood (collected within 72 hours), blood group as per requirement, blood bag number and blood group cross-checked	
4.	Keeps blood at room temperature if blood warmer is not available	
5.	Aspirates stomach contents before the procedure	
6.	Holds the baby's leg and hands in position with a cotton drape	
7.	Cleans the procedure area and drapes with three sterile sheets so that only the umbilical area is visible	
8.	Ties the gauze piece at the base of the umbilicus loosely	
9.	Cuts the umbilicus is cut at 1 cm above the base with the clean surgical blade	
10.	Identifies the umbilical vein at 11 o'clock position	
11.	Cannulates the umbilical vein with a pre-saline-filled umbilical catheter attached to three-way cannula	
12.	Connects the transfusion set and IV set properly	
13.	Starts cycle with pull out and pushes in same volume	
14.	Monitors hemodynamic during the procedure	
15.	Sends the last aliquot for packed cell volume (PCV), total serum bilirubin (TSB)	
16	Writes the procedure notes	
17.	Discards the waste in an appropriate color bag	
	Total (17)	

Endotracheal Intubation

■ OBJECTIVE

The participants should be able to perform endotracheal intubation in neonates safely and efficiently.

■ SUPPLIES

- Two pairs of sterile gloves
- Disposable ET tubes (size 2.5–4.0 mm internal diameter)
- New batteries (AA/AAA size): Two in number
- Straight blade laryngoscope with blade sizes 00, 0, and 01 with batteries
- Bulb for laryngoscope
- Scissors
- Cut tapes for holding the tube in position.
- Bag and mask with reservoir and oxygen tubing
- Suction catheters (8–10F) and suction machine

■ STEPS

- Gather the supplies (**Fig. 1**).
- Ensure you have a person to assist and help you.
- Wash hands and put on sterile gloves.
- Place the neonate on a flat surface, with head in midline and neck slightly extended by a shoulder roll.
- Ensure that pulse oximeter is attached to the right upper limb.

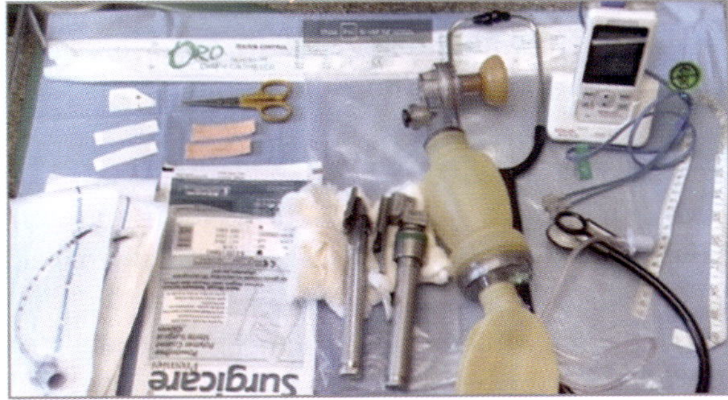

Fig. 1: Gather all the supplies.

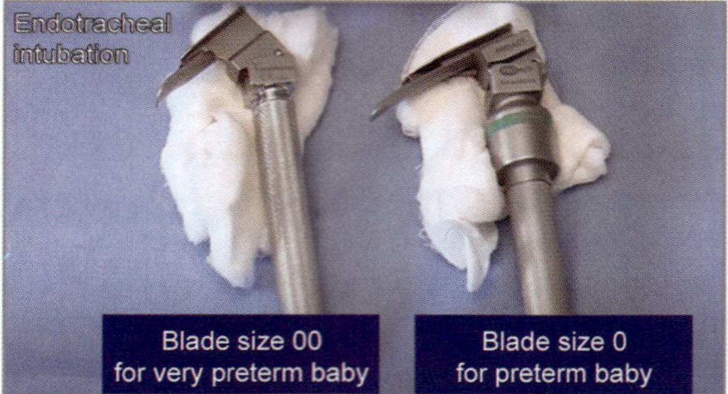

Fig. 2: Size of laryngoscope blades.

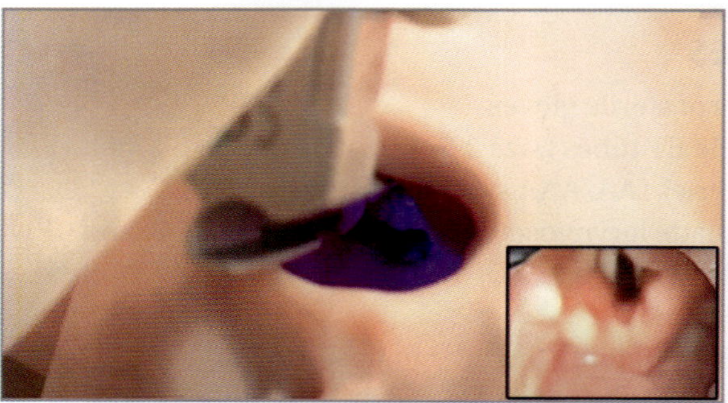

Fig. 3: Slide the laryngoscope over the tongue with tip of
blade resting on vallecula

- Ensure positive pressure ventilation has been given and SpO_2 before attempting intubation is above 95%.
- Choose the appropriate size blade of laryngoscope (0 for preterm and 00 for very preterm neonate) **(Fig. 2)**.
- Choose the appropriate size endotracheal tube
- <1,000 g/<28 weeks: 2,5 mm; 1,000–2,000 g/28–34 weeks: 3.0 mm; 2,000–3,000 g/35–38 weeks: 3.5 mm and for >3,000 g/>38 weeks: 3.5–4.0 mm
- Hold the laryngoscope in left hand and stabilize the infant's head with right hand.
- Slide it over the tongue with the tip of blade resting on vallecula.
- Lift the blade slightly lifting the tongue out of the way to visualize pharyngeal area **(Fig. 3)**.
- Clear the secretions as needed.
- Visualize the epiglottis, insert the ET tube sliding it along the side of tongue till the tube enters between vocal cord and up to black band (vocal cord guide) **(Fig. 4)**.
- Remove laryngoscope while firmly holding against baby's palate.
- Hold the tube against the baby's palate.
- Administer positive pressure ventilation (PPV).

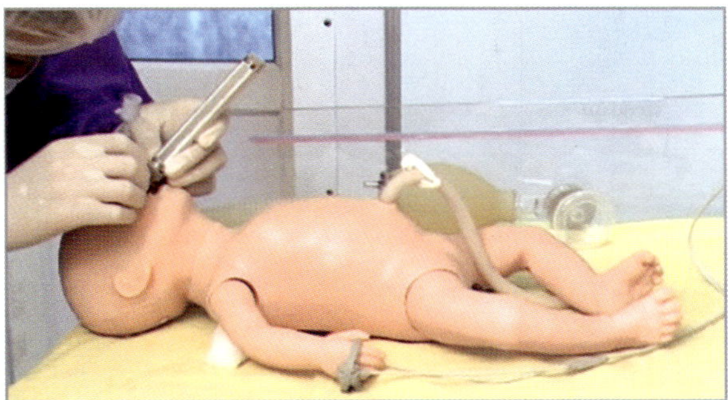

Fig. 4: Slide the ET tube along side of tongue.

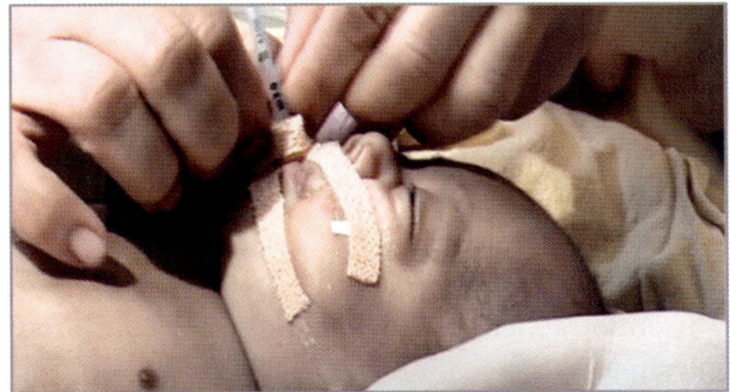

Fig. 5: Secure the tube by tape to upper lip.

- Observe symmetrical chest movements.
- Assistant should check for bilateral chest movement, air entry in axilla and rising heart rate.
- If the chest is not moving, remove the endotracheal tube and resume PPV by bag and mask.
- Repeat intubation, observe chest movement and assistant should again check for air entry and heart rate.
- Assistant should check the distance from tip to lip to be correct (using nasotragal length)
- Secure the tube by tape to upper lip **(Fig. 5)**.
- Continue positive pressure ventilation.
- Cut the endotracheal tube approximately 4 cm beyond the lip to reduce the dead space **(Fig. 6)**.
- Document the procedure with date, time, and indication of intubation.
- Discard the biomedical waste in appropriate color-coded bag.

DO'S

- Always call for help and ensure there is an additional person to help and assist you

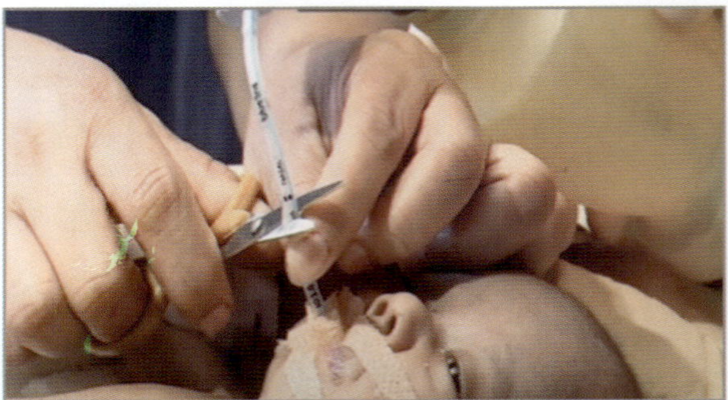

Fig. 6: Cut the endotracheal tube to reduce the dead space.

- Keep monitoring the vitals (Heart rate and SpO_2) throughout the procedure and switch to bag and mask ventilation in case of deteriorating vitals.
- Do keep a watch for complications of intubation such as hypoxia, bradycardia, apnea, and pneumothorax.

■ DON'TS ⊗

- The tip of the endotracheal tube, which is the key part, should NOT touch any unsterile area.
- Do not take >30 seconds for attempting intubation. Continue bag and mask ventilation before reattempting.
- No role of free flow oxygen in the procedure; use bag and mask ventilation if the baby gasps or there are worsening vitals.
- Do not use rocking movements while introducing the endotracheal tube.
- No need for shortening the length of the tube.

■ FURTHER READING

1. Deorari AK. Practical Procedures for the Newborn Nursery. 5th edition. 2018.
2. IAP NNF Neonatal Resuscitation (chrome-extension://efaidnbmnnnibpca-jpcglclefindmkaj/https://iapindia.org/pdf/Ch-104-Neonatal-Resuscitation-Program.pdf last accessed 20th March 2024)
3. Newbornwhocc.org. Preterm care package. Available from: https://youtu.be/H26p4HY-1Q8 [Last accessed March, 2024].

TABLE 1: Objective structured clinical examination (OSCE) for endotracheal intubation.

S. No.	Steps	Points (1 each)
1.	Gathers the supplies	
2.	Ensures that there is an additional person to assist and help	
3.	Washes hands and puts on sterile gloves	
4.	Places the neonate on a flat surface, with head in midline and neck slightly extended by a shoulder roll	
5.	Ensures that pulse oximeter is attached to right upper limb	
6.	Ensures positive pressure ventilation has been given and SpO_2 before attempting intubation is above 95%	
7.	Chooses the appropriate size blade of laryngoscope (0 for preterm and 00 for very preterm neonate)	
8.	Chooses the appropriate size endotracheal tube <1,000 g/<28 weeks: 2,5 mm; 1,000–2,000 g/28–34 weeks: 3.0 mm; 2,000–3,000 g/35–38 weeks: 3.5 mm and for >3,000 g/>38 weeks: 3.5–4.0 mm	
9.	Holds the laryngoscope in left hand and stabilizes the infant's head with right hand	
10.	Identifies the landmarks and takes corrective action to visualize glottis	
11.	Inserts tube from right side without obstructing the vision	
12.	Aligns vocal cod guide with vocal cords.	
13.	Removes laryngoscope while firmly holding against baby's palate	
14.	Holds the tube against the baby's palate	
15.	Administers positive pressure ventilation (PPV)	
16.	Observes for symmetrical chest movements	
17.	Assistant checks for bilateral chest movement, air entry in axilla and rising heart rate	
18.	If the chest is not moving, remove the endotracheal tube and resume PPV by bag and mask	
19.	Assistant checks the distance from tip to lip to be correct (using nasotragal length)	
20.	Secures the tube by tape to upper lip	
21.	Continues positive pressure ventilation	
22.	Documents the procedure with date, time, and indication of intubation	
23.	Discards the biomedical waste in appropriate color-coded bag	
	Total (23)	

Endotracheal Suction

■ OBJECTIVE

The participants should be able to do endotracheal suction in ventilated neonates, safely and efficiently. The purpose of the suctioning is to remove secretions accumulated around the tip and within the lumen of endotracheal tube.

■ SUPPLIES

- Two pairs of sterile gloves
- Sterile suction catheter
- Suction tubing and collection canister
- Sterile water to clear catheter and tubing
- Resuscitation bag
- Tape measure.

■ STEPS

- Gather the supplies.
- Wash hands and put on sterile gloves.
- Suction should be performed only if clinically indicated.
- Determine the size of suction catheter to be inserted. (5–6 Fr for 2.5 mm ET, 6 Fr for 3.0 mm and 8 Fr for >3.0 mm size ET).
- Determine the depth of insertion for the suction catheter by noting the centimeter mark at the lip and then measuring the distance from the lip to the end of ET adaptor. Add the two numbers together **(Figs. 1 to 3)**.
- The suction catheter should be inserted not >0.5 cm past the end of ETT (endotracheal tube) or damage to the airway may result.
- Chart the suction catheter size to be used and suction catheter depth on the ETT card at the bedside for future use.
- Lay the measuring tape on the bed.
- Adjust the negative pressure gauze on wall suction to 80–100 mm Hg **(Fig. 1)**.
- Attach the suction catheter to suction tube, holding it in the sterile gloved hand **(Fig. 2)**.
- Ensure that the tip of the suction catheter, which is the key part, should not touch any unsterile area around the baby.

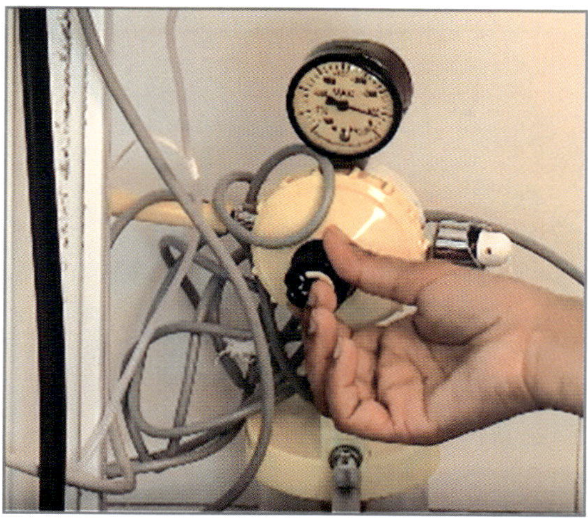

Fig. 1: Adjust the suction pressure on the wall suction.

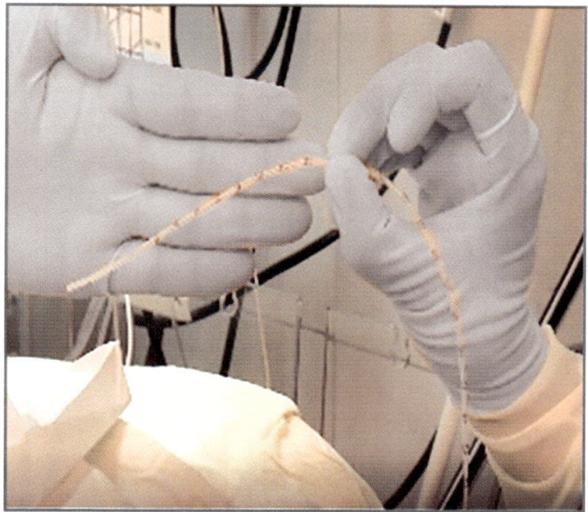

Fig. 2: Hold the suction tube in the sterile gloved hand.

- Monitor the vitals and note the heart rate, respiratory rate, and oxygen saturation **(Fig. 4)**.
- Monitor the SpO_2 with the pulse oximeter and increase the FiO_2 by 10–20% if there is desaturation.
- Insert the suction catheter to the predetermined length.
- Apply negative pressure as the catheter is withdrawn at no more than a 5-second period.
- Slowly rotate the catheter out.
- Put back the neonate on ventilator within 20 seconds and allow time to recover.
- Repeat the steps 13 to 17 if needed.

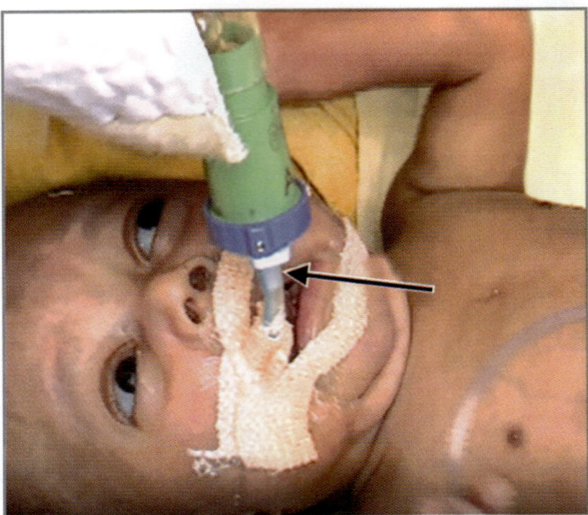

Fig. 3: Measure the tip of the ET to the adapter end.

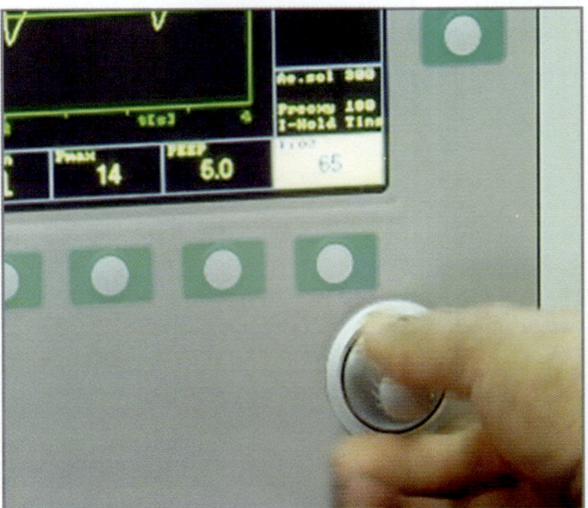

Fig. 4: Attach the monitor for vitals.

- It may be needed to pass the catheter 2 to 3 times to clear the airway.
- If needed, 0.2 mL normal saline may be instilled, and five ventilator breaths allowed before suctioning a neonate with thick secretions **(Fig. 5)**.
- Suction the oral cavity followed by nasal cavity after doing ET suction, to remove any accumulated secretions, either with same catheter or using a separate 8F–10F suction catheter if needed.
- It may be necessary to increase the ventilatory settings (PIP, rate, and oxygen) before the baby returns to pre-suction status.
- Gradually decrease the FiO_2 to pre suction level.
- Assess and note the type of secretions from ET.

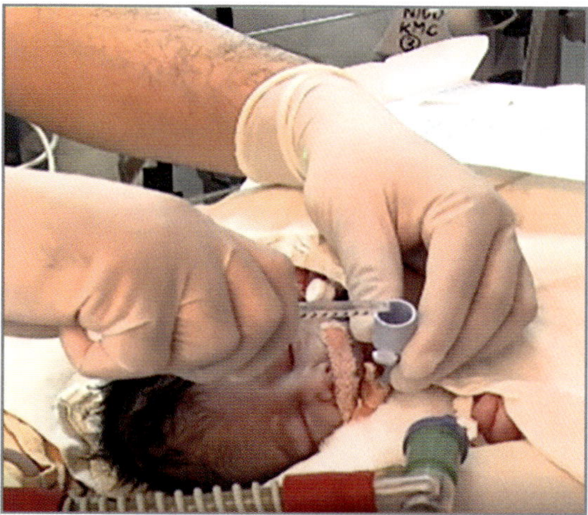

Fig. 5: If need be, instill normal saline.

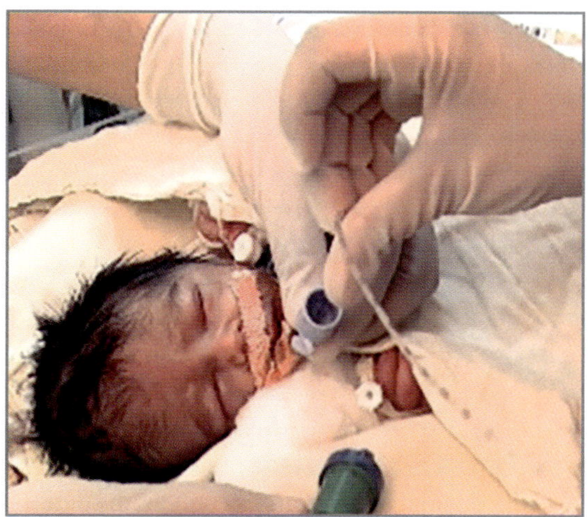

Fig. 6: Suction the oral cavity followed by nasal cavity after ET suction.

- Monitor the vitals and auscultate bilateral air entry.
- Discard the catheter after single use in the appropriate color-coded bag **(Fig. 7)**.
- Document the procedure in clinical notes.

■ DO'S ✅

- Always follow strict asepsis while ET suctioning, since it is potential source of ventilator-associated pneumonia in case of any breach in asepsis.
- Keep monitoring the vitals before, during and after the procedure **(Fig. 8)**.
- Suction only when clinically indicated (some common indications are visible secretions, changes in breath sounds, desaturations).

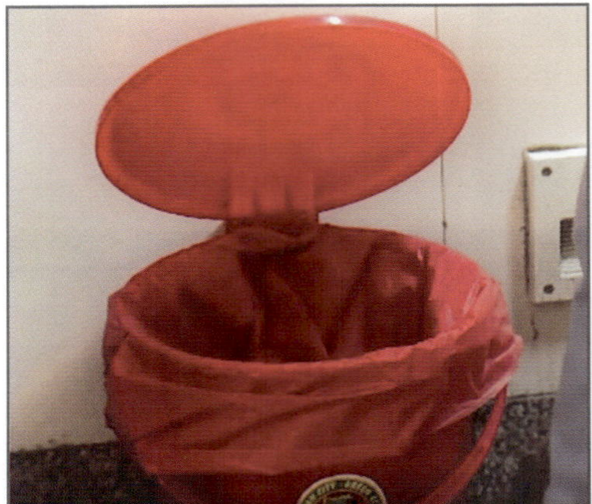

Fig. 7: Discard the catheter in appropriate color coded bag.

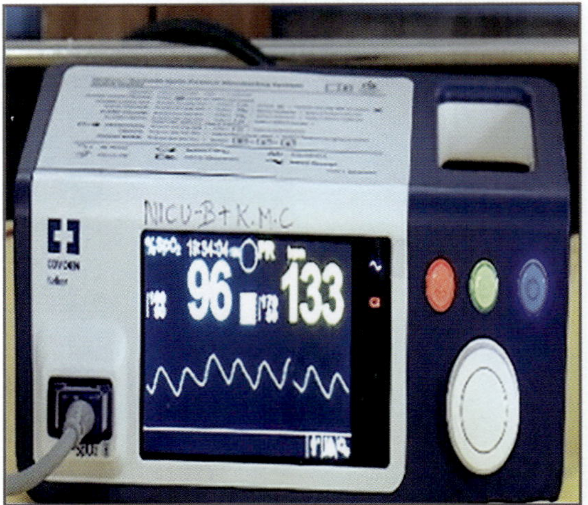

Fig. 8: Keep monitoring the vitals throughout the procedure.

■ DON'TS

- Do not allow the tip of suction catheter, which is the key part, to touch any unsterile surface.
- Do not insert the suction catheter beyond the predetermined length since we should not hit the carina or enter the bronchus while suctioning.

■ FURTHER READING

1. Deorari AK. Practical Procedures for the Newborn Nursery. 5th edition. 2018.
2. Newbornwhocc.com. Common preterm care package. Available from: https://youtu.be/rv_b0be0f7Q [Last accessed March, 2024].
3. Newbornwhocc.org. Facility based preterm care package; 2017.

TABLE 1: Objective structured clinical examination (OSCE) for endotracheal suctioning (in ventilated neonates).

S. No.	Steps	Points (1 each)
1.	Gathers the supplies	
2.	Washes hands and puts on sterile gloves	
3.	Determines the need for suctioning; it should be performed only if clinically indicated	
4.	Determines the size of suction catheter to be inserted. (5–6 Fr for 2.5 mm ET, 6 Fr for 3.0 mm and 8 Fr for >3.0 mm size ET)	
5.	Determines the depth of insertion for the suction catheter by noting the centimeter mark at the lip and then measuring the distance from the lip to the end of ET adaptor. Add the two numbers together. The suction catheter should be inserted not >0.5 cm past the end of ETT or damage to the airway may result	
6.	The suction catheter should be inserted not >0.5 cm past the end of ETT or damage to the airway may result	
7.	Charts the suction catheter size to be used and suction catheter depth on the ETT card at the bedside for future use	
8.	Lays the measuring tape on bed	
9.	Adjusts the negative pressure gauze on wall suction to 80–100 mm Hg	
10.	Attaches the suction catheter to suction tube, holding it in the sterile gloved hand	
11.	Monitors the vitals and note the heart rate, respiratory rate, and oxygen saturation	
12.	Inserts the suction catheter to the predetermined length	
13.	Applies negative pressure as the catheter is withdrawn at no more than a five-second period	
14.	Slowly rotates the catheter out	
15.	Puts back the neonate on ventilator within 20 seconds an allow time to recover	
16.	Indicates that it may be needed to put the catheter 2–3 times to clear the airway	
17.	Tells that if needed, 0.2 mL of normal saline may be instilled, and five ventilator breaths allowed before suctioning a neonate with thick secretions	
18.	Suctions the oral cavity followed by nasal cavity after doing ET suction, to remove any accumulated secretions, either with same catheter or using a separate 8F–10F suction catheter if needed	
19.	Assesses and notes the type of secretions from ET	
20.	Monitors the vitals and auscultate bilateral air entry after the procedure	
21.	Discards the catheter after single use in the appropriate color-coded bag	
22.	Documents the procedure in clinical notes	
	Total (22)	

Surfactant Administration Via Insure

■ OBJECTIVE

The participants should be able to administer surfactant via INSURE technique safely and efficiently.

■ SUPPLIES (FIG. 1)

- Two pairs of sterile gloves
- 5-mL syringe
- Feeding tube 6F or 5F
- Sterile blade/scissors
- Surfactant vial
- Laryngoscope with appropriate size blades (size 00 and 0)
- ET tube (2.5 or 3 as appropriate)
- T piece resuscitator or self-inflating bag
- Oxygen and air source
- Cardio-respiratory monitoring equipment

■ STEPS

- Gather the supplies.
- Wear cap and mask.

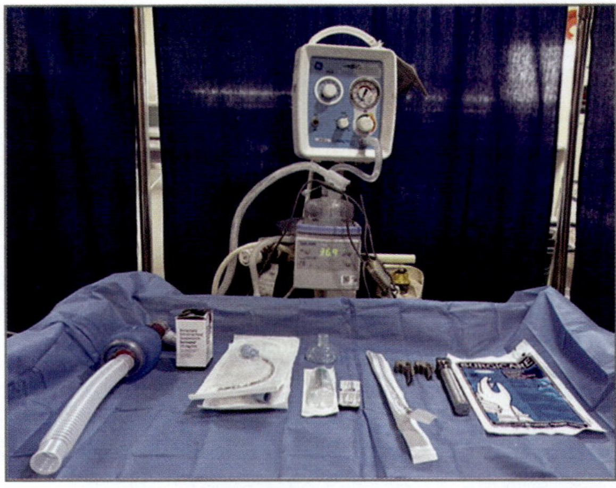

Fig. 1: Equipment required for INSURE.

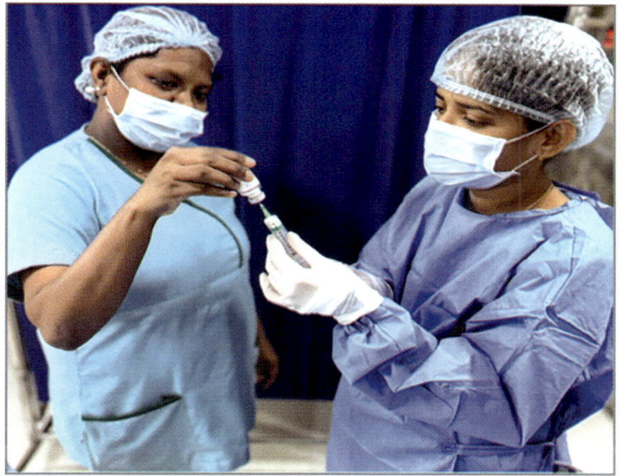

Fig. 2: Drawing desired amount of surfactant.

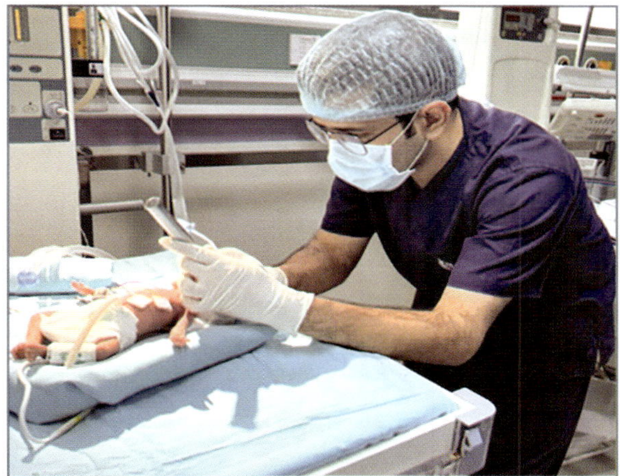

Fig. 3: Intubate with appropriate size ET tube.

- Wash hands and put on sterile gown and gloves.
- Premedicate with caffeine if required.
- Draw the required amount of Surfactant into syringe using large bore needle **(Fig. 2)**.
- Measured required length of feeding tube and cut in sterile manner (total length of ET tube and 3 cm for adapter) **(Fig. 3)**
- Discontinue CPAP, intubate the baby with appropriate size ET tube.
- Insertion length 0.5–1 cm below vocal cord (measured depth: nasotragal length + 1 cm)
- Confirm the ET position by auscultation.
- Continuous monitoring with pulse oximeter for heart rate and saturation.

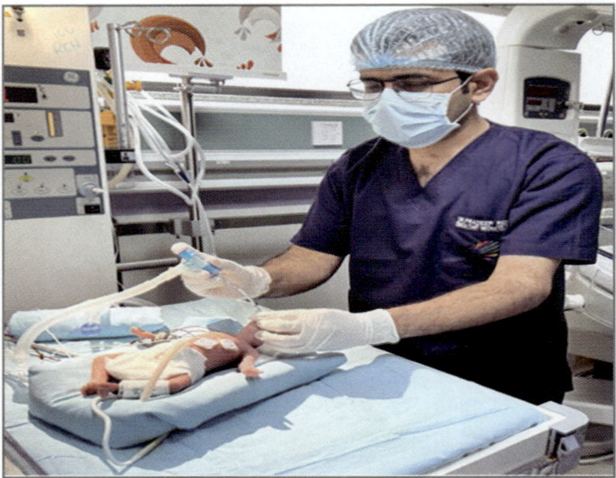

Fig. 4: Positive pressure ventilation as required.

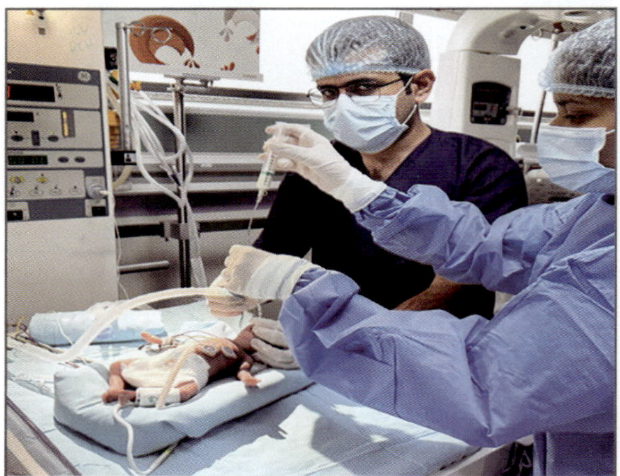

Fig. 5: Administration of surfactant in 2–3 aliquots.

- Administration of surfactant 100–200 mg/kg in 2–3 aliquots over 1–3 minutes depending upon volume using precut feeding tube **(Figs. 3 to 5)**.
- Provide positive pressure ventilation (PPV) in between aliquots with longer inspiratory time (Ti) **(Fig. 6)**.
- Push 1 cm of air to flush the catheter.
- Extubate the baby and continue on CPAP after the procedure **(Fig. 7)**.
- Discard the waste in wastebin.
- Wash hands and document the procedure.

■ DO'S ✅

- Follow nonpharmacological pain relief measures such as swaddling.

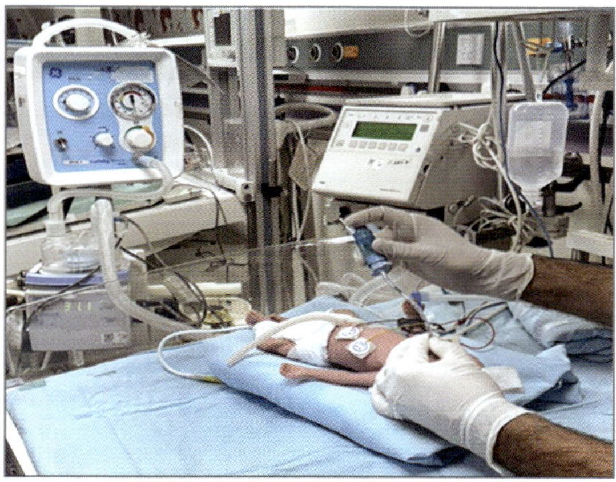

Fig. 6: Positive pressure ventilation with T piece in-between the aliquots.

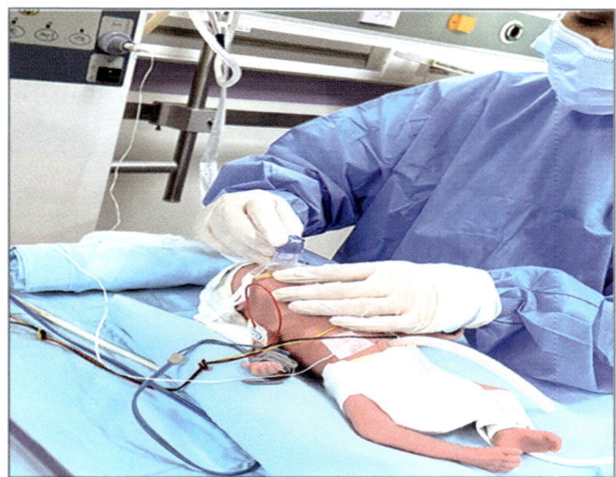

Fig. 7: CPAP—post-extubation following surfactant administration.

- Provide adequate positive pressure ventilation in between surfactant administration.
- Monitor Vitals (RR, HR, and Saturations) throughout the procedure.

■ DON'TS ❌

- Avoid sedation.

■ FURTHER READINGS/TO WATCH

1. https://www.newbornwhocc.org/2019_pdf/Surfactant%20Replacement%20 Therapy%20%20-%202019.pdf
2. YouTube. Available from: https://youtu.be/rCkpMXg2m4A [Last accessed March, 2024].
3. YouTube. Available from: https://youtu.be/mGLCdrM6q0A [Last accessed March, 2024].
4. YouTube. Available from: https://youtu.be/jPdVmmaybXw [Last accessed March, 2024].

TABLE 1: Objective structured clinical examination (OSCE) for surfactant administration—INSURE method.

S. No.	Steps	Points (1 each)
1.	Washes hands	1
2.	Gathers the supplies	1
3.	Attaches to cardiorespiratory monitor (i.e., pulse oximeter) for monitoring	1
4.	Measured required length of feeding tube and cut in sterile manner	1
5.	Calculation of insertion depth of ET tube	1
6.	Calculation of surfactant dose	1
7.	Draws the required amount of the surfactant into syringe and connect to feeding tube	1
8.	Non-pharmacological measures for pain relief	1
9.	Intubation with appropriate size ET tube	1
10.	Checks the position of the ET tube	1
11.	Administration of surfactant in 2–3 aliquots	1
12.	Positive pressure ventilation with T piece in-between the aliquots	1
13.	CPAP—Post-extubation following surfactant administration	1
14.	Monitors vitals (RR, HR, and saturations) throughout the procedure	1
15.	*Documentation of procedure*	1

Surfactant Administration Via Thin Catheter (Less Invasive Surfactant Administration/Minimally Invasive Surfactant Therapy)

■ OBJECTIVE

The participants should be able to administer surfactant via thin catheter safely and efficiently.

■ SUPPLIES

- Two pairs of sterile gloves
- 5-mL syringe
- Feeding tube 6F or commercially available surfactant catheter
- Surfactant vial (prewarmed to room temperature)
- Laryngoscope (preferably video laryngoscope).

■ STEPS

- Gather the supplies.
- Wear cap, mask.
- Wash hands and put on sterile gown and gloves.
- Increase CPAP pressure by 1–2 cmH$_2$O and elevate head end by 15–20°.
- Identify a helper to help in monitoring and to attach the syringe containing surfactant.
- Intratracheal insertion of thin catheter or feeding tube using direct laryngoscopy.
- Insertion depth 0.5–1 cm beyond vocal cords (measured depth: nasotragal length + 1 cm) **(Fig. 1)**.
- Continuous monitoring with pulse oximetry for heart rate and saturation.
- Administration of surfactant (phospholipid 100–125 mg/kg) in 1–2 aliquots over 1–3 minutes depending upon volume **(Figs. 2 and 3)**.
- Pause if desaturation or bradycardia <100 beats/minute is observed.
- Push 1 cm of air to flush the thin catheter.
- CPAP pressure back to previous levels 10–15 minutes after the procedure.
- Discard the waste in wastebin.
- Wash hands and document the procedure.
- Postprocedure monitoring for bradycardia, desaturation or apnea.

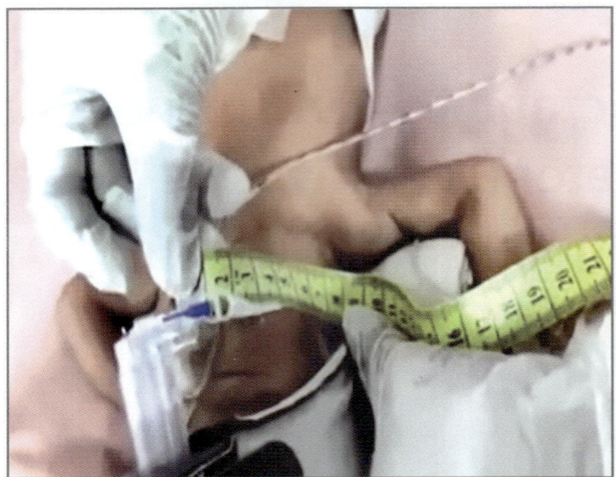

Fig. 1: Measurement using Nasotragal length +1 cm.

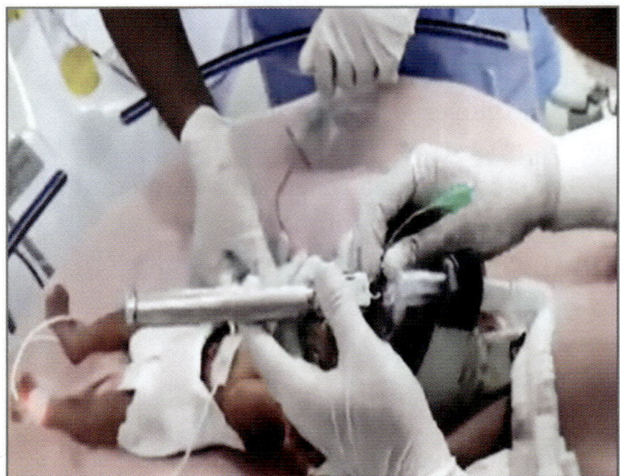

Fig. 2: Administration of surfactant in 2 to 3 aliquots.

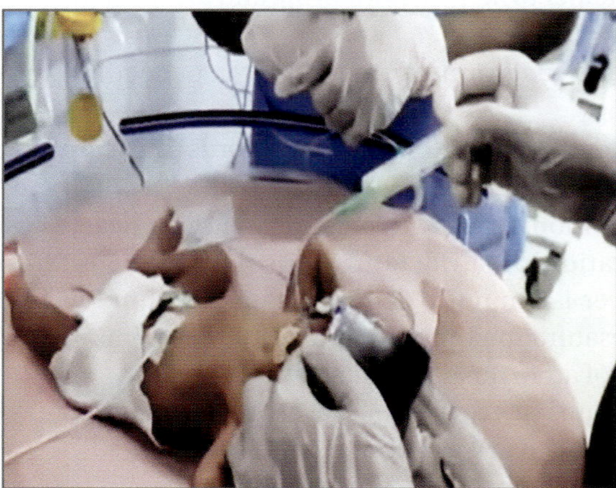

Fig. 3: Administration of surfactant in 2 to 3 aliquots.

■ DO'S ✓

- Follow nonpharmacological pain relief measures such as swaddling.
- Atropine and fentanyl may be used in select cases.
- Remove laryngoscope after insertion of thin catheter.
- Watch for bradycardia, desaturation during and after procedure.
- Use an objective scale such as Silverman Anderson score to assess and monitor progression of respiratory distress.

■ DON'TS ✗

- Do not disconnect CPAP during the procedure.
- Do not use suction for 4–6 hours after administration of surfactant.
- No role of change of posture during and after procedure.

■ FURTHER READING

1. Bellos I, Fitrou G, Panza R, Pandita A. Comparative efficacy of methods for surfactant administration: a network meta-analysis. Arch Dis Child Fetal Neonatal Ed. 2021;106(5):474-87.
2. Devi U, Pandita A. Surfactant delivery via thin catheters: methods, limitations, and outcomes. Pediatr Pulmonol. 2021;56(10):3126-41.
3. Panza R, Laforgia N, Bellos I, Pandita A. Systematic review found that using thin catheters to deliver surfactant to preterm neonates was associated with reduced bronchopulmonary dysplasia and mechanical ventilation. Acta Paediatr. 2020;109(11):2219-25.

TABLE 1: Objective structured clinical examination (OSCE) for LISA.

S. No.	Steps	Points (1 each)
1.	Wash hands	1
2.	Gather the supplies	1
3.	Calculation of insertion depth	1
4.	Attaching pulse oximeter for monitoring	1
5.	Calculation of surfactant dose	1
6.	Nonpharmacological measures for pain relief	1
7.	Removing laryngoscope after insertion of thin catheter	1
8.	Documentation of procedure	1

Ventilator-associated Pneumonia Prevention Bundle Checklist

Bundle approach is a set of evidence-based practices which are expected to improve patient outcomes. Individual elements of bundles are protocolized well established practices. The whole team must agree collectively and implement them reliably.

TABLE 1: "Ventilator Associated Pneumonia" Prevention bundle.

S. No.	Steps	Step performed (Yes/No)
Hand hygiene		
1.	Wash hands with soap and water	
2.	Wear mask, cap, and gloves	
3.	Do not touch baby or baby's environment with gloves	
4.	Handwash or hand rub after removing gloves	
Endotracheal tube care		
1.	During intubation, aseptic technique is to be maintained, mask and gloves to be worn	
2.	Oral intubation to be preferred than nasal	
Humidification		
1.	Heated humidifier is a must	
2.	Inspired gas at 37°C and 100% relative humidity	
3.	Always use auto-refill technique for the humidifier to fill water	
4.	No condensation in inspiratory limb	
5.	Drain condensate in water trap	
6.	Consider condensate as an infectious waste and discard accordingly	
Respiratory equipment care		
1.	Ventilator circuits and oxygen therapy equipment should be readily available	
2.	Ventilator circuits should be used only once if disposable, and if reusable they should be sterilized after each use, as per unit disinfection and sterilization protocol	

Contd...

Contd...

S. No.	Steps	Step performed (Yes/No)
3.	Ventilator circuits should be changed when visible soiled	
4.	The respiratory care equipment should be handled under strict asepsis	
5.	Endotracheal suction should be done preferably by two health personnel with one person assisting in handling the suction catheter aseptically	
6.	CPAP system should not be allowed to be standby for >12 hours	
7.	Resuscitation bags not to be kept on bed, but they have to be hung outside the warmers	
8.	Resuscitation bags should be replaced once a week	
9.	The circuit to be positioned parallel to the baby and in a dependent position	
Position of infant		
1.	30–45° elevation of head end	
2.	Lateral decubitus is the preferred position	
3.	Frequent changes in position	
Stress ulcer prophylaxis		
1.	Acidic gastric content prevents bacterial contamination	
2.	Avoid using antacids such as ranitidine	
Oral hygiene		
1.	Oral suction to prevent pooling of secretions	
2.	Moisten the lips with saline	
3.	Avoid reusable suction tubes for oral suction	
4.	Chlorhexidine oral application is optional	
Enteral feeds		
1.	Encourage oral feeds through the orogastric tube	
2.	Prefer EBM over formula	
3.	Trophic feeds if not on enteral feeds	
Shorter duration of intubation and ventilation (Intubation and extubation to be done strictly as per unit protocol)		
1.	Daily consideration of extubation readiness on morning rounds and shift to noninvasive mode of ventilation as early as possible	
2.	Sedation vacation for all neonates who are on sedation	
3.	Consider use of noninvasive ventilation in the first place	

Contd...

Contd...

S. No.	Steps	Step performed (Yes/No)
4.	Wean off invasive ventilation as soon as possible	
5.	Prevent unplanned extubation	
6.	Avoid unnecessary reintubation	
Post-extubation		
1.	Frequent change in position (as indicated clinically)	
2.	Oral and nasal suction as indicated clinically	
3.	Nebulization SOS	
4.	Watch for respiratory distress. (signs of respiratory distress in ventilated neonates, which include increased work of breathing, subcostal or intercostal retractions, irritable on ventilator, reduced SpO_2)	
Continuing training and audits		
	Regular training of healthcare professionals	
	Re-enforcement of hand hygiene practices in the unit	
	Regular audits of the checklists	

Oral Suction (in Nonventilated Neonates)

◼ OBJECTIVE

The participants should be able to do safe and effective oral suction in non-ventilated neonates. The purpose of the suctioning is to remove secretions from the oral and nasopharyngeal area of the nonintubated neonate using catheter to ensure airway patency and to prevent aspiration of oral or gastric secretions.

◼ SUPPLIES

- Two pairs of sterile gloves **(Fig. 1)**.
- Suction catheter 5 or 6 FG for preterm, 8 FG for term neonates **(Fig. 2)**.
- Wall suction/portable suction machine **(Fig. 3)**.
- Sterile water/normal saline **(Fig. 4)**.

◼ STEPS

- Collect supplies.
- Wash hands and don sterile gloves.
- Attach the appropriate size catheter to suction tubing.
- Occlude the catheter completely and set pressure on suction to 100 mm Hg (130 cmH$_2$O).
- Estimate the length of the catheter to be inserted by measuring from the tip of the nose to the tip of ear lobe **(Fig. 5)**.

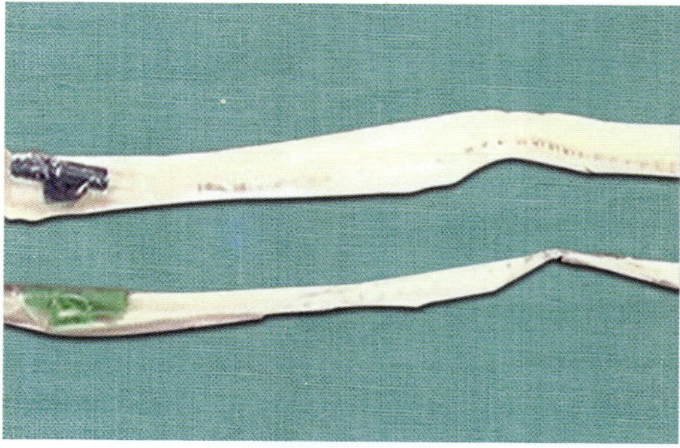

Fig. 1: Appropriate size suction catheter.

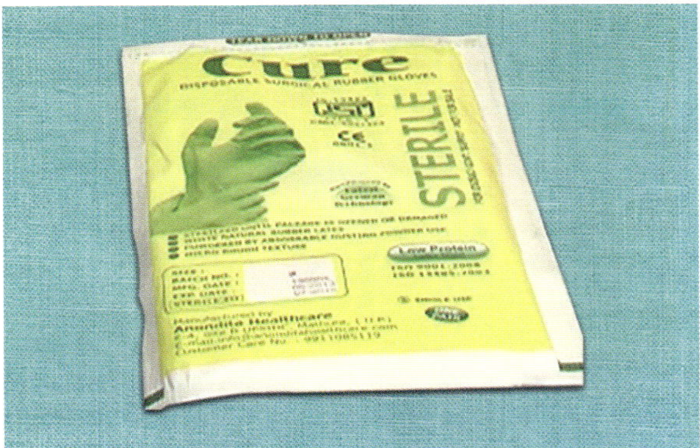

Fig. 2: Appropriate size suction catheter.

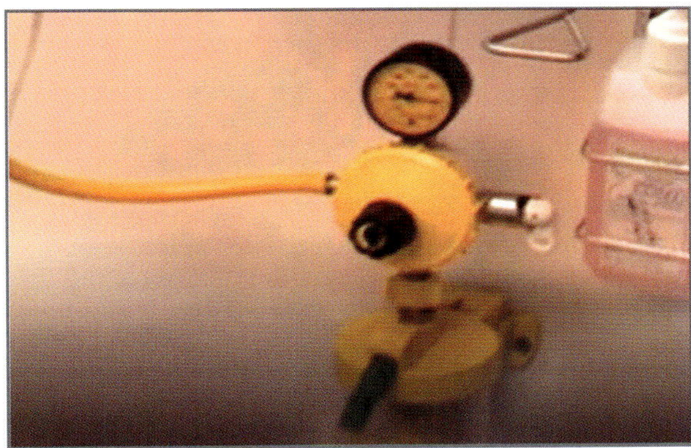

Fig. 3: Suction machine.

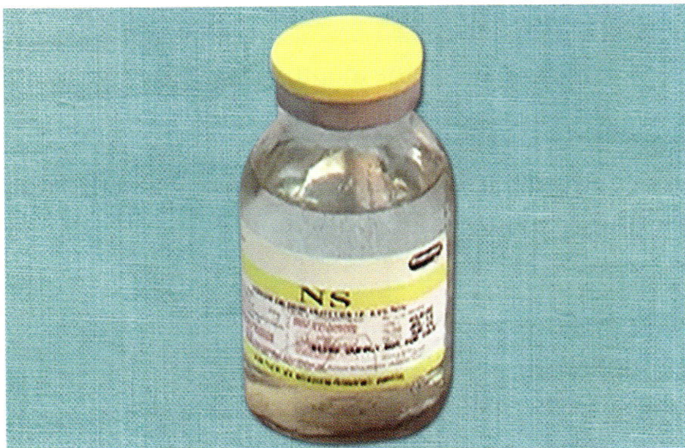

Fig. 4: Normal sline.

- Gently insert the catheter to the measured distance from the mouth.
- The direction of catheter insertion should be upward and backward.
- Apply suction only upon withdrawal of catheter (limit attempts to 3–5 seconds or less).

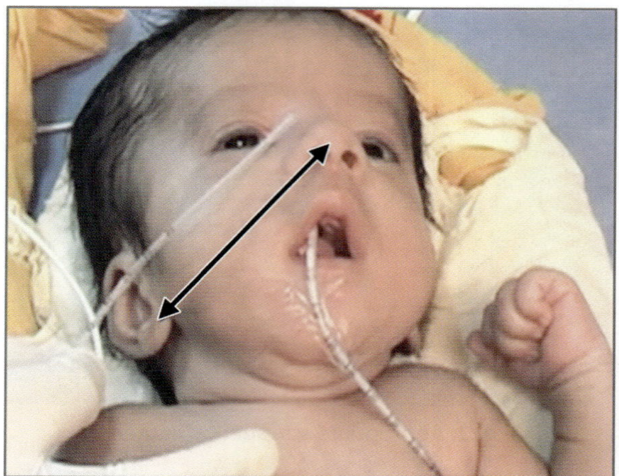

Fig. 5: Measure the suction catheter.

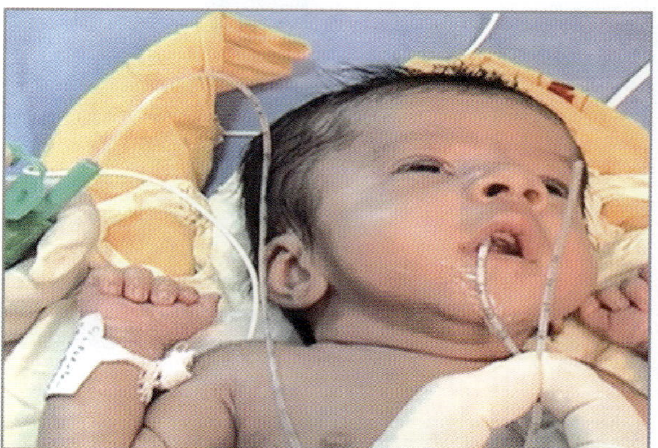

Fig. 6: Suction the mouth before the nose.

- Reposition the infant after doing suction.
- Discard the catheter after single use in an appropriate bag as per biomedical waste management guidelines.

■ DO'S ✓

- Try a smaller catheter if the catheter is difficult to pass.
- Limit attempts to 3–5 seconds or less.
- Monitor the vitals before and during the procedure, watch for bradycardia
- Suction mouth prior to nares to reduce the risk of gasping aspiration **(Fig. 6)**.

■ DON'TS ✗

- Do not allow the tip of suction catheter, which is the key part, to touch any unsterile surface **(Fig. 7)**.

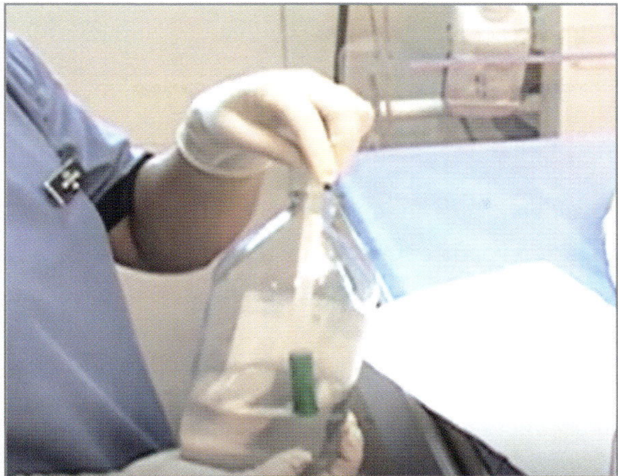

Fig. 7: Do not allow the tip of suction catheter to touch external surfaces

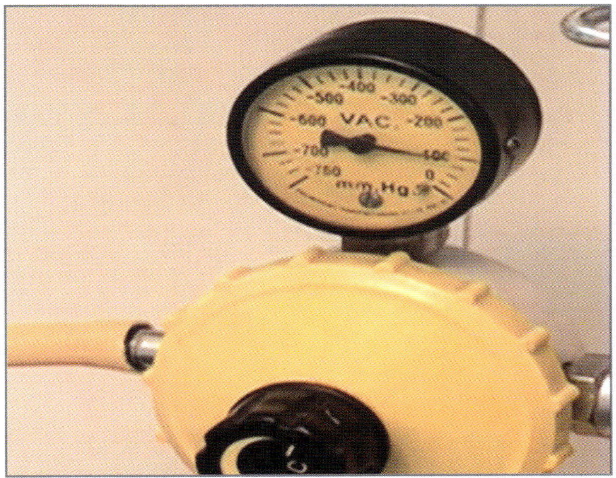

Fig. 8: Do not exceed the pressure beyond recommended range to avoid trauma.

- Do not use excessive pressure as it may cause mucosal trauma **(Fig. 8)**.
- Do not pass the catheter completely through the nares to clear secretions as it may cause trauma.
- If the neonate is on CPAP/NIPPV (continuous positive airway pressure/ nasal intermittent positive pressure ventilation), do not disconnect the CPAP/NIPPV interface, while nebulizing. Use hood box to provide adequate mist around the nose.

■ FURTHER READING

1. Facility-Based Care of Preterm Infant. Available from: https://www.pretermcare-eliminatingrop.com/index.php [Last accessed March, 2024].
2. https://youtu.be/oUFwRBgpJ_Y (videos on common neonatal procedures by newbornwhocc.org)

S. No	Steps	Points (1 each)
TABLE 1: Objective structured clinical examination (OSCE) for oral suction (in nonventilated neonates).		
1.	Gathers the supplies	
2.	Washes hands and puts on sterile gloves	
3.	Attaches the appropriate size catheter to suction tubing	
4.	Occludes the catheter completely and set pressure on suction to 100 mm Hg (130 cmH$_2$O)	
5.	Estimates the length of the catheter to be inserted by measuring from the tip of the nose to the tip of ear lobe	
6.	Gently inserts the catheter to the measured distance from the mouth	
7.	Inserts suction catheter gently upwards and back into nares	
8.	Applies suction only upon withdrawal of catheter (limit attempts to 3–5 seconds or less)	
9.	After suctioning, repositions the infant	
10.	Discards the catheter after single use in appropriate color coded bag as per biomedical waste management	
	Total (10)	

24 CHAPTER

Blood Product Transfusion in Neonates

■ OBJECTIVE

To know how to use blood product judiciously and safely.

■ SUPPLIES

- Peripheral intravenous (IV) line insertion tray
- Blood group bag to be transfused and cross-checked
- Infusion pump
- Blood transfusion set
- Keep few pedipacks to reduce multiple donor exposure for multiple transfusion.

■ STEPS

- Check the indication of transfusion of blood product.
- Informed consent from the parents
- Check neonates' blood group and blood group on the bag.
- Details on the blood product to be checked for patient ID
- Check ID of the patient, both should correspond.
- Document the volume to be transfused in the case sheet with rate of infusion and bag details.
- Put peripheral IV line and initiate transfusion with all aseptic precaution.
- Document the blood transfusion procedure and details of the bag on the patient's file.
- Monitoring of vital parameter during transfusion.
- Document the completion of the procedure in patient's records.

■ DO'S

- Strictly follow the guidelines for blood transfusions.
- Platelet transfusion should be always cross-matched and should be given immediately (30 minutes).
- Stop maintenance fluid, unless treated for hypoglycemia.
- Use of pedipacks reduces donor exposure for multiply transfused preterm.
- A blood count should be performed 1 hour and 24 hours after completion of the transfusion, in order to evaluate the efficacy of the transfusion.

■ DON'T'S 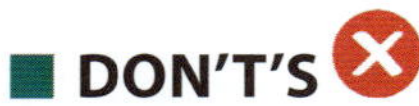

- Routinely withhold feeding during transfusion unless hemodynamically unstable.
- Give diuretics routinely after blood transfusion.

■ CHECKLIST FOR BLOOD TRANSFUSION

Blood transfusion	Yes	No
Before transfusion:		
Look for indication of transfusions		
Check all the supplies		
Informed consent taken from parents		
Check patients' details identification and blood product		
Check for neonates' blood group and blood product		
Document the volume to be transfused with rate		
Take extra sample for further workup		
During transfusion:		
Put peripheral IV line with all aseptic precautions		
Look for any local site reactions		
Monitor vitals [heart rate (HR), respiratory rate (RR), peripheral oxygen saturation (SpO$_2$), perfusion] during transfusion		
Check the amount of blood component left as lime elapsed		
Document completion of the procedure on the patients' records		
After transfusion:		
Monitoring should be continued post transfusion for 2–4 hours		
Total (13)		

■ FURTHER READING

1. Franz AR, Engel C, Bassler D, Rüdiger M, Thome UH, Maier RF, et al; ETTNO Investigators. Effects of Liberal vs Restrictive Transfusion Thresholds on Survival and Neurocognitive Outcomes in Extremely Low-Birth-Weight Infants: The ETTNO Randomized Clinical Trial. JAMA. 2020;324(6):560-70.
2. New HV, Berryman J, Bolton-Maggs PH, Cantwell C, Chalmers EA, Davies T; British Committee for Standards in Haematology. Guidelines on transfusion for fetuses, neonates and older children. Br J Haematol. 2016;175:784-828.
3. Whyte R, Kirpalani H. Low versus high haemoglobin concentration threshold for blood transfusion for preventing morbidity and mortality in very low birth weight infants. Cochrane Database Syst Rev. 2011;11:CD000512.

Central Lines in Neonate

Performing Umbilical Venous and Arterial Catheterization

■ OBJECTIVE

The participants should be able to cannulate/catheterize umbilical venous or/and arterial access.

■ SUPPLIES

- Umbilical catheter size 3.5 F or 5.0 F
- Scalpel (blade no.) **(Fig. 1)**
- Curved iris forceps
- 3-0 silk and needle
- Three-way stopcock
- 5 mL syringe
- 0.9% normal saline
- Sterile gauze
- Heparinized saline (10 U/mL)
- Disinfectant (e.g., Chlorhexidine 0.5%)
- Tape
- Manikin for umbilical access

> *UAC—single lumen:*
> <1.2 kg—3.5 Fr
> >1.2 kg—5 Fr
>
> *UVC—single or double:*
> <3.5 kg—5 Fr
> >3.5 kg—8 Fr

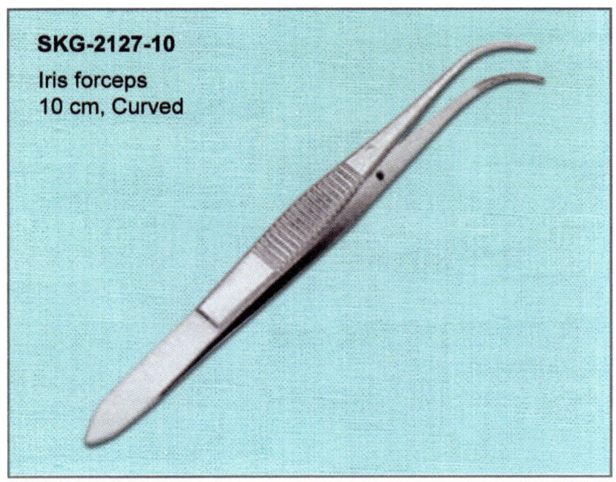

Fig. 1: Curved iris forceps.

■ STEPS

- Document about any local infection/signs of NEC and bruising of lower extremities and/or feet and toes prior to placement.
- Hand washing and followed by maximal sterile barrier
- All catheters must be attached to appropriate stopcock or syringe, flushed, and filled with normal saline before insertion to avoid air emboli.
- Drape around the umbilical stump with sterile towels, taking care not to obscure infant's face and upper chest.
- Tie a cord tie to prevent bleeding, but not so tight as to block passage of the catheter.
- Cut the cord horizontally about 1–1.5 cm from the skin (**Figs. 2 and 3**).
- Identify vessel to be cannulated and immobilize cord.

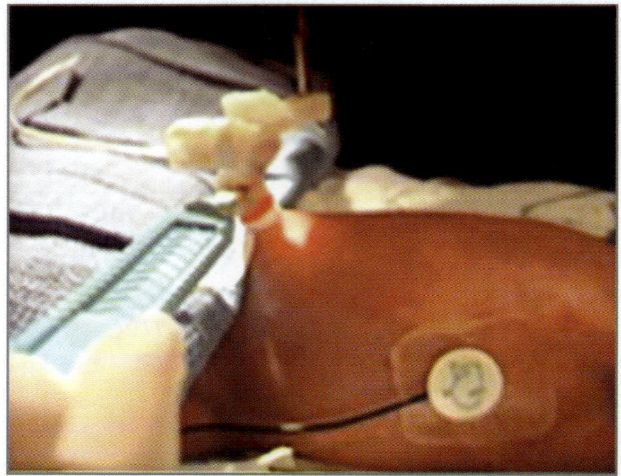

Fig. 2: Cut the cord horizontally about 1 to 1.5 cm from the skin.

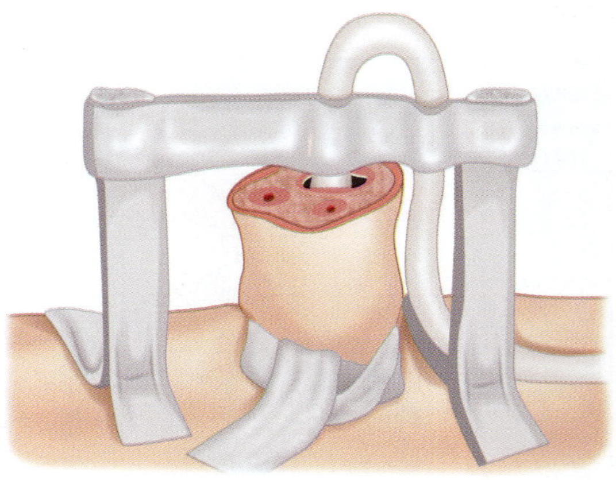

Fig. 3: Umbilical venous catheterization.

Umbilical Artery Cannulation

INSERTION TECHNIQUE AND ESTABLISHING THE UAC LINE

- Using iris forceps, one of the two arteries is dilated.
- Insert one point of curved iris forceps into lumen up to 0.5 cm and probe gently.
- Remove forceps, bring both points together and reintroduce probe gently. Allow points to spring apart and maintain in this "open" position about 15 seconds to dilate artery.
- Grasp the catheter 1 cm from tip by hand or with curved forceps and insert into dilated lumen.
- Advance with a firm steady motion; mild upward traction of cord toward head of infant while advancing may facilitate passage of catheter
- After advancing catheter about 5 cm verify intraluminal position by checking for easy withdrawal of blood and "pulsation" of blood/saline in the catheter, then clear with flush solution.
- Advance umbilical artery cannulation (UAC) to the predetermined length.
- After dilation, a 3.5–5 Fr catheter attached to a three-way stopcock flushed with normal saline solution (without heparin) is inserted into the artery.
- Central umbilical artery access requires advancement of the catheter to either a low or high position. A low line lies just above the aortic bifurcation between the 3rd and 4th lumber vertebrae, and a high line lies above the diaphragm between the 6th and 9th thoracic vertebrae.
- To determine the optimal position for high or low catheter locations, use formulas or graphs (*see* **Figures 4 and 5**) or beside ultrasonography (USG) may be used.
- Add low-dose heparin (0.5–1.0 U/mL) to the fluid infused through the UAC. A commonly used solution is 0.45% NaCl with 0.5–1 IU heparin/mL running at 1 mL/h.
- Securing the catheter to the abdominal wall using a "bridge/goal post" method of taping **Figure 3**.
- Optimal duration of a UAC line is 5–7 days.

INSERTION TECHNIQUE AND ESTABLISHING THE UAC LINE

The umbilical vein is the larger and thinner-walled of the vessels and is usually at the 11 to 12 o'clock position.

- Gently insert tips of iris forceps into lumen of vein to remove any clots.
- Introduce flushed, normal saline (NS)-filled umbilical venous catheter (UVC) and advance to predetermined length.

UAC distance (cm) = Birth weight (kg) × 3 + 9

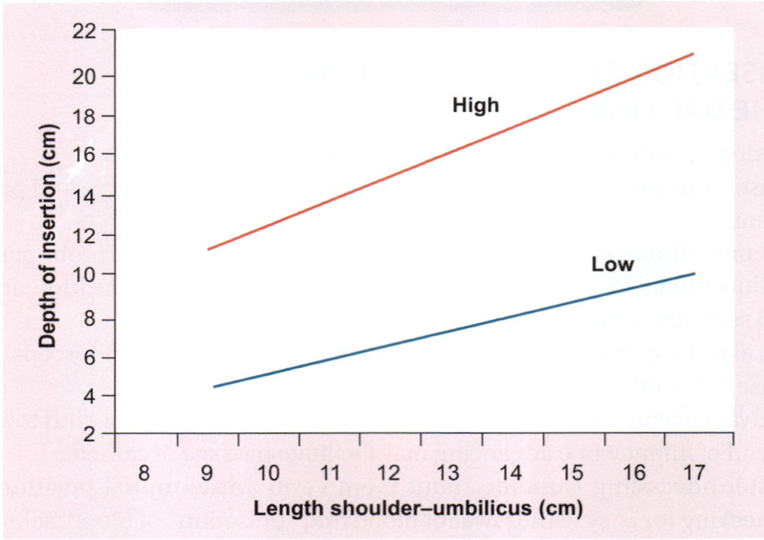

Fig. 4: Umbilical artery cannulation (UAC) distance.

UVC length (cm) = 3 × birth weight (kg) + 9/(2 + 1)

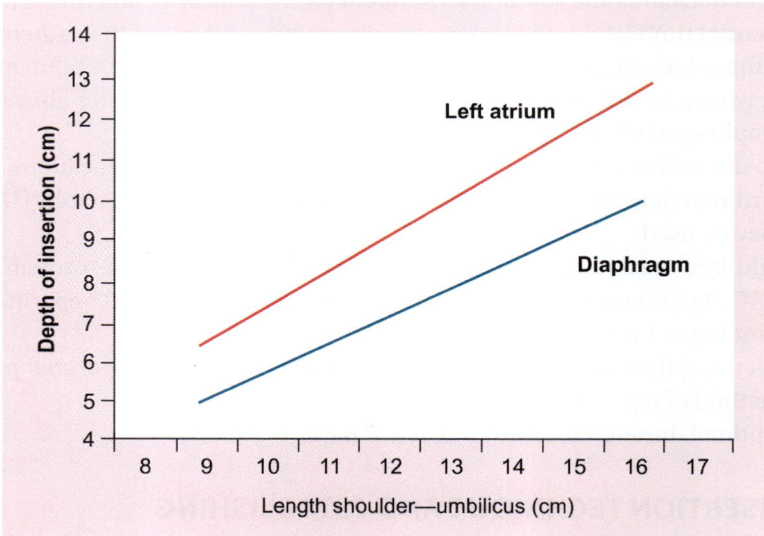

Fig. 5: Umbilical venous catheter (UVC) length.

- Direct the catheter cephalad or toward the head as the vein lies in this direction.
- For resuscitative measures, as in a cardiac or respiratory arrest, an umbilical vein is only cannulated to approximately 2–4 cm beyond

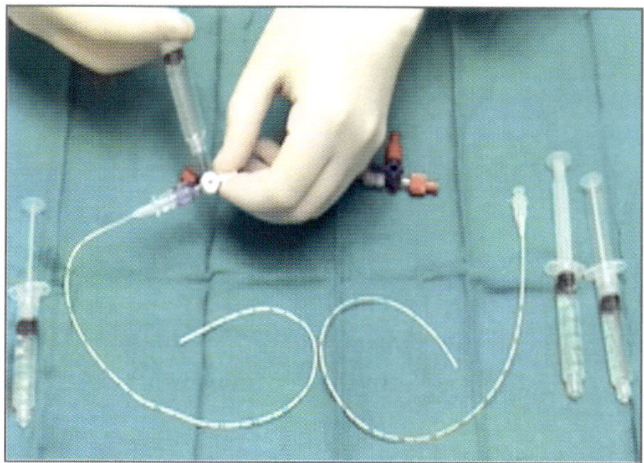

Fig. 6: Insert the flushed catheter and dont leave open to air to avoid thrombu.

the mucocutaneous junction and only until adequate blood return is obtained.

- In nonemergencies, the catheter is advanced until it is in the inferior vena cava just below the level of the right atrium.
- Do not leave the catheter open to atmosphere as there is a danger of air emboli **(Fig. 6)**.
- There is little data to support the use of UVC heparinization.
- Optimal duration of a UVC line is 5–7 days.

Peripherally Inserted Central Catheter

■ OBJECTIVE

The participants should be able to cannulate/catheterize device inserted into a peripheral vein and threaded into the central venous circulation.

■ SUPPLIES

- Restraints or swaddling device (optional)
- *Catheter equipment:*
  - 1.1–2 F (28- to 23-gauge) catheter, with sufficient length to achieve appropriate catheter tip placement for infants weighing <2,500 g
  - 1.9–3 F (26- to 20-gauge) catheter, with sufficient length to achieve appropriate catheter tip placement for infants weighing ≥2,500 g
- Nontoothed forceps

■ PROCEDURE FOR PICC INSERTION IN AN INFANT

- Determine need for a PICC (peripherally inserted central catheter)
- Obtain informed consent (as per hospital protocol)
- Select the vein to be used for the procedure
  - Use in the following order to have less complication
  - UL > LL
  - Right side > Left side (right more direct to central circulation)
  - Basilic vein > cephalic vein (basilic larger than cephalic and less tortuous
- The following veins are used for PICC insertion in neonates:
  - *Veins of arms:* Basilic and median cubital basilica vein, axillary vein
  - *Scalp and neck:* External jugular, temporal and posterior auricular
  - *Vein of legs:* Femoral, saphenous, and popliteal vein
- Measure the length of the catheter to be inserted **(Figs. 1 and 2)**.

■ STEPS

- *Preparation of catheter:* Flush catheter, attach a 10-mL syringe, (never use 1–2 mL syringe because it can create high pressure leading to rupture of catheter) to the catheter.
- Position the patient and restrain as needed.
- *Arm insertion:* Abduct the arm to a 90° angle, with the patient's head turned toward the arm.

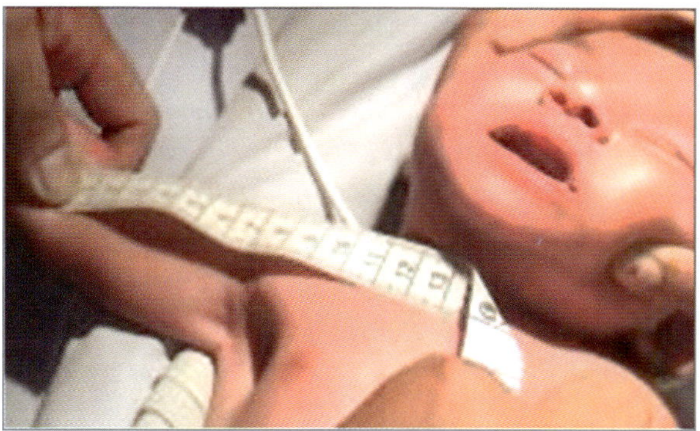

Fig. 1: Measure from the insertion site along the course of the vein, to the right of the sternal border, to the third intercostal space. If insertion is through an arm vein, extend the arm at a 90° angle for measuring.

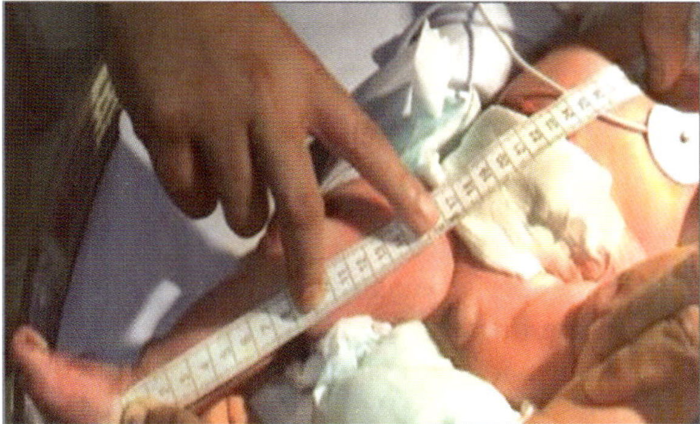

Fig. 2: *Lower limb:* Measure from the insertion site along the course of the vein, to the right of the umbilicus and up to the xiphoid.

- *Axillary vein insertion:* Abduct the arm 100°–130° or place the infant's hand by the head and puncture parallel and inferior to the artery.
- *Femoral vein insertion:* Position the infant "frog-legged"; insert the introducer at a 30° angle 1 cm below the inguinal ligament and 5 mm medial to the femoral pulse.
- Insert the introducer bevel up at a 15°–30° angle into the skin a few millimeters before anticipated entry into the vein. Hold the skin taut below the level of insertion to prevent the vein from rolling. A 30° angle is recommended for insertion into the femoral vein.
- When the vessel is cannulated, observe for blood return (blood return may be observed or a "pop" may be felt).
- Using nontoothed forceps, thread the catheter through the introducer needle in 0.5–1 cm increments to the premeasured length.
- To facilitate insertion, flush with saline while threading the catheter if obstruction is realized.

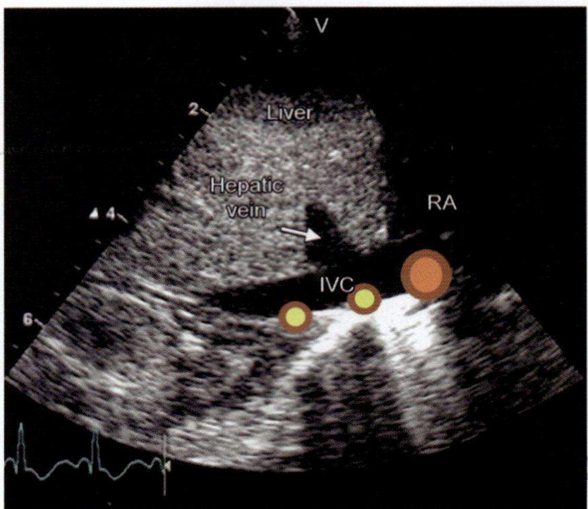

Fig. 3: Inferior vena cava (IVC): Sagittal view.

- If a stylet is present, remove it slowly over a period of 30–60 seconds.
- Aspirate for a blood return and flush the catheter.
- Keep the catheter patent by flushing it intermittently with 0.5 mL flush solution in a 5–10 mL syringe.
- *Catheter tip:* Near superior vena cava (SVC) (if upper limb) OR Inferior vena cava (IVC) near diaphragm (if using lower limb).
- Use sterile semitransparent dressing.

ULTRASOUND ASSESSMENT OF UVC POSITION

- Ideal location of UVC to minimize complication is outside the heart at the IVC/RA (right atrial) junction.
- On chest X-ray (CXR) this may correspond to T9–T10, just above right hemidiaphragm but below the heart.

ULTRASOUND VIEWS

- *Standard views:*
  - Subcostal–parasagittal view **(Fig. 3)**
  - Parasternal short axis view
  - Apical four chamber view
  - Modified views
- Parasternal short axis toward xiphoid

CENTRAL VENOUS CANNULATION

Central venous cannulation (CVC) involves percutaneous placement of a vascular catheter with its tip in the lumen of a major, high-flow vein of the abdomen, or thorax.

STEPS

- Aseptic technique (use maximum sterile barrier)
- Catheter kit with intravascular catheter, finder needle, flexible guidewire, saline solution and syringes, 3 or 5 mL, silk suture (3.0 or 4.0), needle holder
- *Monitoring:* Pulse oximeter, cardiac monitor, blood pressure monitor
- *Medications:* Lidocaine (1%), midazolam 0.1 mg/kg, and morphine sulfate 0.1–0.15 mg/kg, oxygen, suction, airway
- *Appropriate site selection:* To decrease infection risk: prefer internal jugular vein (IJV) > femoral vein
- *Appropriate catheter selection:* Use single lumen catheter
- *Know the anatomy:* Use ultrasonography (USG)

FEMORAL VEIN CANNULATION

Steps

- The lower extremity should be positioned with slight external rotation at the hip and flexion at the knee (frog leg appearance).
- A rolled towel under the buttock may facilitate successful venous access.
- The femoral artery should be located by palpation or ultrasound or in the pulseless patient, assumed to be at the midpoint between the pubic symphysis and anterior superior iliac spine.
- The area over the intended puncture site should be infiltrated with local anesthetic.
- The needle should be inserted 1–2 cm below the inguinal ligament, just medial to the femoral artery, and slowly advanced while negative pressure is applied to a syringe attached to the introducer needle.
- The needle should be directed at a 15°–45° angle toward the umbilicus.
- Once the free flow of venous blood is observed, the syringe should be removed, while the needle is carefully stabilized, and the guidewire is introduced gently.
- After getting it secured with silk suture and apply sterile semitransparent dressing.

INTERNAL JUGULAR VEIN CANNULATION

- Internal jugular catheterization can be achieved via multiple approaches.
- Right-sided approaches are preferred due to potential injury to the thoracic duct on the left side.
- The carotid artery should be palpated, as it lies medial to the internal jugular vein within the carotid sheath.
- For all approaches, the patient should be positioned supine and in a slight (15°–30°) Trendelenburg position, with a roll under the shoulders and with the head turned away from the puncture site.
- After getting it secured with silk suture and apply sterile semitransparent dressing.

Central Line Associated Bloodstream Infections (CLABSI) Prevention Checklist

Bundle approach is a set of evidence-based practices which are expected to improve patient outcomes. Individual elements of bundles are protocolized well-established practices. The whole team must agree collectively and implement them reliably.

S. No.	Steps	Step performed (Yes/No)
Insertion bundle		
1.	Establish a central line kit or cart to consolidate all items necessary for the procedure	
2.	Perform hand hygiene with hospital approved alcohol-based product or antiseptic containing soap, before and after palpating insertion sites and also before and after inserting central line	
3.	Use maximum barrier precautions including sterile gown, sterile gloves, surgical mask, cap, and larger sterile drape	
4.	Disinfect skin with appropriate antiseptic before catheter insertion	
5.	Minimize the number of access points	
6.	Keep connecting ports with UVC/UAC (umbilical venous catheter/umbilical artery cannulation) away from diaper area	
7.	Use either a sterile transparent semipermeable dressing or sterile gauze to cover the insertion site	
8.	Prefer upper limb veins over lower limb veins	
9.	Ensure the catheter tip is at proper position	
10.	No blood stains around the insertion site	
11.	The insertion should preferably be done by a skilled trained health personnel who has assisted at least five catheter insertions before	
12.	The health care personnel should always be assisted by a second person while inserting the catheter	

Contd...

Contd...

S. No.	Steps	Step performed (Yes/No)
Maintenance bundle		
1.	Perform hand hygiene with hospital approved disinfectant before and after changing the dressing	
2.	Evaluate the catheter insertion site daily for signs of infection and dressing integrity	
3.	If the dressing is damp, soiled, or loose, change dressing aseptically and disinfect the skin around the insertion site with an appropriate antiseptic	
4.	Develop and use standardized intravenous tubing set up and changes	
5.	Maintain aseptic technique when changing intravenous tubing and when entering the catheter including "scrub the hub"	
6.	Maintenance bundle card to be displayed on the infant warmer for daily audit	
7.	Any creak in circuit of central line should be done in the presence of two health care personnel to maintain asepsis	
8.	Daily review of catheter necessity with prompt removal when no longer needed	
Hub care bundle		
1.	Cleanse hands with soap and water	
2.	Put on gloves	
3.	Establish sterile field under access port	
4.	Place syringes on edge of sterile field	
5.	Scrub access port with alcohol-based solution/antiseptic being used in the neonatal intensive care unit (NICU) as per protocol, for 15 seconds and allow it to dry (clean outside and on top but not inside)	
6.	Pick up syringe keeping the tip sterile	
7.	Attach the syringe to hub, keeping connections sterile	
8.	Administer flush solution keeping connections sterile	
Removal bundle		
1.	Review the need of the central line daily and remove as early as possible	

Chest Tube Insertion

■ OBJECTIVE

Participants should be able to insert chest tube in neonates safely and effectively for various indications.

■ INDICATIONS

- Evacuation of tension pneumothorax
- Evacuation of significant pleural fluid collection [e.g., chylothorax, postoperative hemothorax, empyema, extravasated fluid from upper limb PICC (peripherally inserted central catheter)].

■ WHEN TO SUSPECT PNEUMOTHORAX

Acute deterioration in ventilated infants, either mechanically ventilation or noninvasive ventilation [CPAP or NIPPV (continuous positive airway pressure or nasal intermittent positive pressure ventilation)].

■ RISK FACTORS OF PNEUMOTHORAX

- Requirement of positive pressure ventilation in delivery room, especially in preterm infants
- History of oligohydramnios leading to pulmonary hypoplasia
- Direct trauma to airway following bronchoscopy
- Inappropriate mechanical ventilation setting leading to barotrauma or volutrauma
- Excessive pressure during CPAP

■ WHEN NOT TO INSERT CHEST TUBE

- Small air or fluid collection in pleural space without hemodynamic compromise
- Pneumomediastinum (as air in mediastinum, not in pleural space)
- Pneumopericardium (air in pericardial space)
- Pericardial effusion (fluid in pericardial space)

■ PERSONNEL

At least two persons are required for the procedure, one doctor and other could be either doctor or nursing staff.

EQUIPMENT

- Sterile gloves, sterile gown, cap, mask for the persons doing the procedure
- Neonatal surgical tray consisting sterile swab/cotton balls, sterile surgical drapes, swab holder, needle holder, scissor, mosquito clamp straight, hemostatic forceps, and towel clips.
- 70% isopropyl alcohol and 5% povidone iodine for antiseptic dressing for term infants. For preterm infants, use 0.5% v/v chlorhexidine instead of povidone iodine.
- Surgical blade (no. 15)
- Thoracostomy tube (polyvinyl chloride chest tube with or without trocar; size 8, 10, 12 Fr); alternatively, pigtail catheter can also be used.
- Multipurpose tubing adaptor for connecting chest tube with collection bag
- Underwater seal drainage bag
- Nonabsorbable silk suture on small cutting needle (4-0)
- Towel roll, semipermeable transparent dressing
- 2% Lignocaine solution for local anesthesia and 24% sucrose (or breast milk, dextrose) orally for analgesia; may need IV fentanyl (1–2 µg/kg) on a case-to-case basis only in mechanically ventilated infants.

PREREQUISITES

- Obtain informed consent
- Put on sterile gloves, cap, mask, and gown after washing hands for 60 seconds
- Provide ventilator support as needed (noninvasive or invasive ventilation)
- Monitor vitals; move probe from the operative site to alternative area (legs, opposite wrist) before the procedure. Electrocardiogram (ECG) leads can also be placed and connected to the monitor.
- Confirm the side for chest tube placement by either X-ray or ultrasonography (USG).
- Estimate the length of insertion for intrathoracic portion of tube (skin incision site to mid-clavicle). Usually, 2–3 cm in a small preterm infant and 3–4 cm in a term infant.
- Provide adequate procedural analgesia.
- Sterile dressing and draping surrounding the site of insertion.

POSITIONING OF THE INFANT

Positioning would be different depending on the indication of chest tube insertion. See **Figure 1** for infant position during pneumothorax drainage and **Figure 2** during pleural fluid drainage.

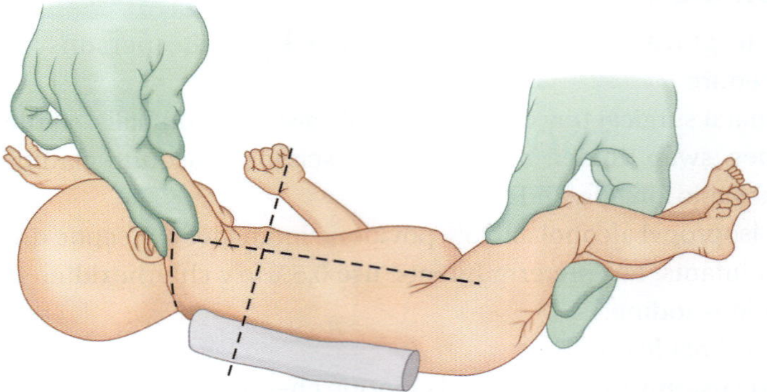

Fig. 1: Affected side up about 60° with the help of a towel roll and arm across the head. This position allows the air to rise up in the thoracic cavity.

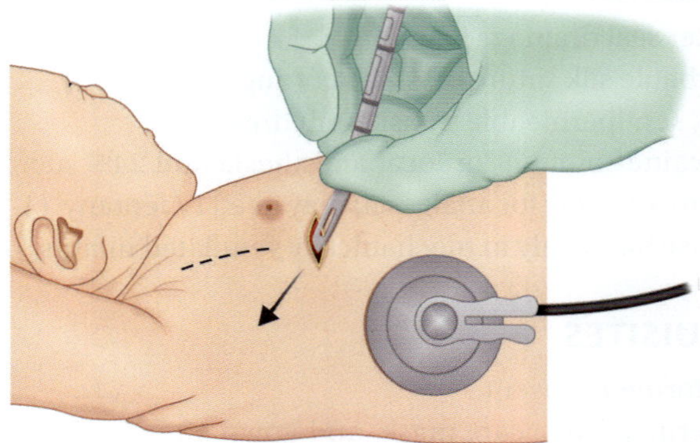

Fig. 2: Supine with slight upward elevation of affected side (150°–30°); arm above the head.

■ POINT OF INSERTION

Incision is made in both scenarios, just above the upper border of lower rib and following the direction of rib:

- *For pneumothorax:* Make an incision (0.5–1 cm) midway between anterior-axillary line (AAL) and midaxillary line (MAL) at fourth intercostal space (ICS) **(Fig. 3)**
- *For pleural collection:* Make an incision (0.5–0.75 cm) just behind the AAL in 6th ICS.

  Be careful to avoid incision of breast tissue by locating the position of nipple and surrounding tissue.

■ SUBSEQUENT STEPS

- Puncture pleura with the tip of a closed hemostatic forceps

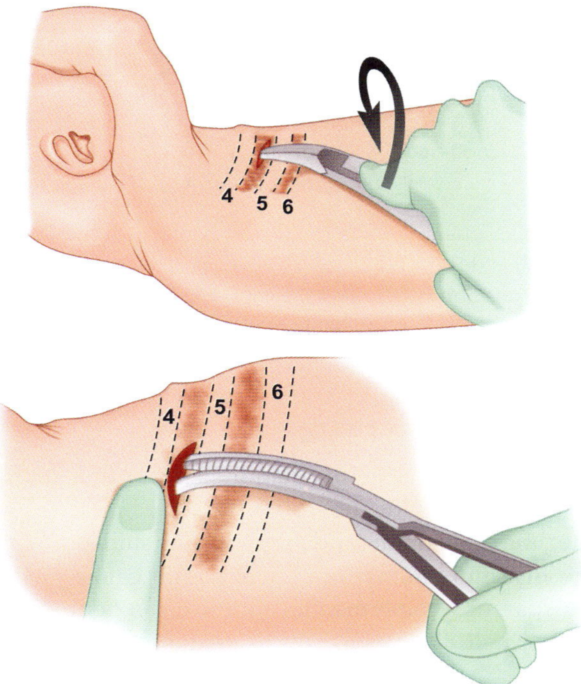

Fig. 3: Point of insertion for pneumothorax.

- A definite "give away" sensation will be felt on puncturing pleura.
- After puncturing pleura open hemostat forceps just enough to pass the chest tube.
- Keeping hemostat in place, and pass the tube between opened tips to the predetermined depth.

ADVANCEMENT AND FINAL POSITION

- Palpate chest wall at the entry site to confirm that the tube is not in the subcutaneous tissue
- *For pneumothorax*: Direct chest tube upward toward apex of thorax and advance tip to midclavicular line, ensuring that all side holes are within the pleural space. Final tip position is in anteromedial pleural space **(Fig. 4)**.
- *For pleural collection*: Insert tube posteriorly only deeply enough to place side holes within pleural space. The final tip position is in posteromedial pleural space **(Fig. 4)**.
- Connect the other end of the chest tube with a multipurpose adaptor and then to the underwater seal drainage with negative pressure of 10–20 cm of water.
- Observe for the movement of the water meniscus in the drainage system.

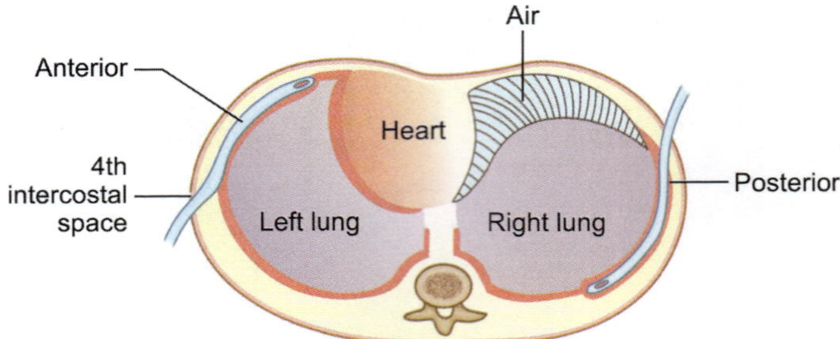

Fig. 4: Anterior tip position in left pleural cavity drains the air effectively. Posterior tip position in right pleural space is unable to evacuate the air, as air collects anteriorly in supine infants.

SECURING THE CHEST TUBE

- Use 4-0 silk suture to close the skin incision with a single interrupted suture on either side of the tube.
- Secure the tube by wrapping and then tying the suture tail around the tube.
- Cover the insertion site with a small sterile gauze piece and a clear, small, transparent semipermeable adhesive. Do not put a large dressing covering the whole chest especially in small preterm infants.

SIGNS OF MALPOSITION OF CHEST TUBE

- Bleeding from the endotracheal tube
- Continuous bubbling in the underwater seal
- No movement of water meniscus in under water seal drainage
- Blood return from the chest tube
- Tube lying neither anterior nor posterior to lung on lateral view
- Tube positioned in fissure (horizontal course towards medial side of lung)
- Persistent pneumothorax despite satisfactory position in anteroposterior (AP) chest X-ray (CXR)
- Increased density around tip of tube in CXR

DO'S

- Provide adequate analgesia by combination of nonpharmacologic and pharmacologic measures.
- While making incision keep away from the breast nodule.
- Make skin incision just above the upper border of lower rib.
- Do an AP and lateral CXR to confirm the tube position and evacuation of air/pleural fluid (**Figs. 5A and B**)
- Adjust ventilatory setting to minimize further air leak
- Always be aware of the signs of malposition
- Watch for the patency of chest tube regularly
- Remove tube at the earliest opportunity

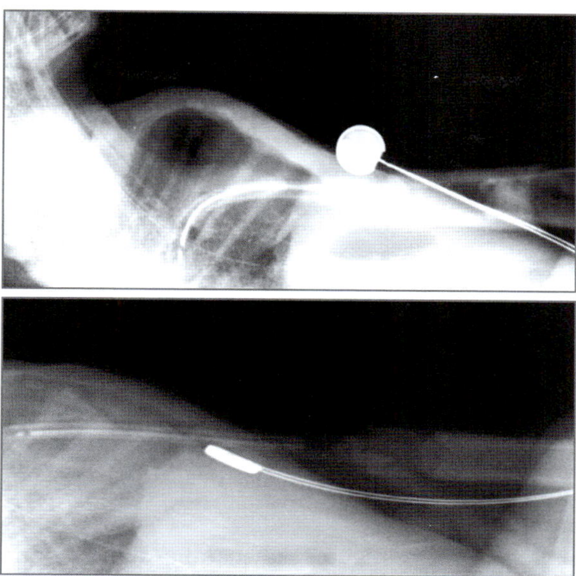

Figs. 5A and B: Importance of doing a lateral chest X-ray (CXR) after chest tube placement. (A) Tip of the tube is directed posteriorly, not able to drain the air and (B) tip of the tube is redirected anteriorly effectively evacuating the pleural air.

■ DON'T'S ✖

- Do not use trocar during tube insertion to avoid visceral injury.
- Do not use trocar to dissect pleura.
- Do not put extensive dressing around the insertion of chest tube.
- Do not put traction on tub.

■ FURTHER READING

1. Markham M. Pulmonary air leak. In: Eichenwald EC, Hansen AR, Martin CR, Stark AR, Jain N (Eds). Cloherty and Stark's Manual of Neonatal Care. South Asian edition. New Delhi: Wolter Kluwer (India); 2021. pp. 482-9.
2. Rais-Bahrami K, MacDonald MG. Thoracostomy. In: MacDonald MG, Ramasethu J, Rais-Bahrami K (Eds). Atlas of Procedures in Neonatology, 5th edition. Philadelphia: Lippincott Williams & Wilkins, Wolters Kluwer; 2013. pp. 255-72.
3. Spruill CT, LaBrecque MA, Upadhyay A. Preventing and treating pain and stress among infants in the newborn intensive care unit. In: Eichenwald EC, Hansen AR, Martin CR, Stark AR, Jain N (Eds). Cloherty and Stark's Manual of Neonatal Care. South Asian edition. New Delhi: Wolter Kluwer (India); 2021. pp. 1061-82.
4. Weiner GM, Zaichkin J. Lesson 10: Special consideration. Textbook of Neonatal Resuscitation, 8th edition. USA: American Academy of Pediatrics; 2021. pp. 243-63.

Use of Nebulizer

■ OBJECTIVE

The participants should be able to use nebulizer for neonates, safely, and efficiently.

■ SUPPLIES

- Two pairs of sterile gloves
- Nebulizing chamber
- Mouthpiece or mask
- Tubing to attach the gas inlet on the chamber to either an air or oxygen supply
- Oxygen hood
- Medication to be administered (in appropriate dilution)

■ STEPS

- Gather the supplies **(Fig. 1)**.
- Wash hands and put on sterile gloves.
- Ensure that the nebulizer is clean/sterilized appropriately.

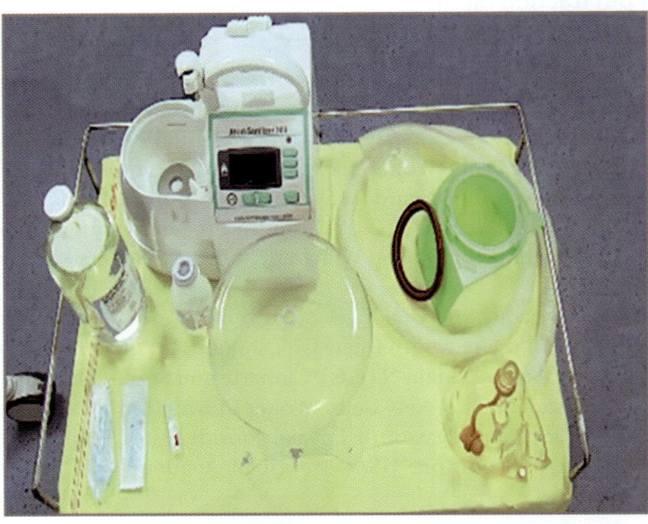

Fig. 1: Gather all the supplies.

- Keep the neonate supine and maintain comfort.
- Measure the exact dose of medication to be administered and pour into the nebulizing chamber.
- Add saline to make volume up to 2–4 mL.
- Connect the nebulizer to the electric source.
- Connect the nebulizer tubing to port on the compressor.
- Select the appropriate size oxygen mask to connect to the mouthpiece.
- Monitor the vitals before starting the nebulizer.
- Switch on the nebulizer.
- Hold the nebulizer in upright position to avoid spillage while using the mask and ensure that it fits well.
- Start oxygen at 4–6 L/min.
- Nebulize till no aerosol is seen and nebulizer sounds empty.
- Document the medication given and its dose and note if any side effects (oxygen saturation, etc.).

■ DO'S ✔

- Ensure that the parts of nebulizer are clean before each use.
- Use saline, not distilled water for dilution to avoid reflex bronchospasm.
- Discard the residual solution since residual solution can get colonized rapidly with bacteria from environmental sources.
- Wash the three parts of nebulizer with soap and water.
- Monitor the vitals before and after nebulization. Look for adverse effects like tachycardia **(Fig. 2)**.
- Do clean the filter (in ultrasonic nebulizer) regularly to prevent dust accumulation.

■ DON'TS ✖

- Do not use chlorhexidine-based solutions for cleaning

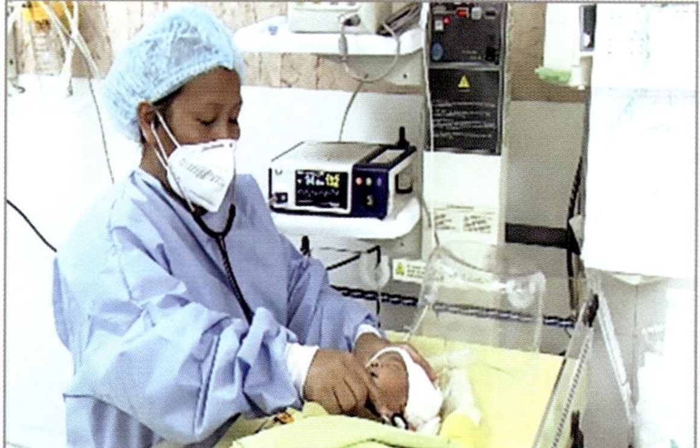

Fig. 2: Monitor and record vital signs and breath sounds before nebulization.

- Do not use the nebulization chamber if any signs of (1) discoloration, (2) stickiness, and (3) cracking of chamber.
- If the neonate is on CPAP/NIPPV (continuous positive airway pressure or nasal intermittent positive pressure ventilation), do not disconnect the CPAP/NIPPV interface, while nebulizing. Use hood box to provide adequate mist around the nose.

■ FURTHER READING

1. https://youtu.be/oUFwRBgpJ_Y (videos on common neonatal procedures by newbornwhocc)

TABLE 1: Objective structured clinical examination (OSCE) for nebulizer use.

S. No	Steps	Points (1 each)
1.	Gathers the supplies	
2.	Washes hands and puts on sterile gloves	
3.	Ensure that the nebulizer is clean/sterilized appropriately	
4.	Keep the neonate supine and maintain comfort	
5.	Measure the exact dose of medication to be administered and pour into the nebulizing chamber	
6.	Add saline to make volume up to 2–4 mL	
7.	Connect the nebulizer to the electric source	
8.	Connect the nebulizer tubing to port on the compressor	
9.	Select the appropriate size oxygen mask to connect to the mouthpiece	
10.	Monitor the vitals before starting the nebulizer	
11.	Switch on the nebulizer	
12.	Hold the nebulizer in upright position to avoid spillage while using the mask and ensure that it fits well	
13.	Start oxygen at 4–6 L/min	
14.	Nebulize till no aerosol is seen and nebulizer sounds empty	
15.	Document the medication given and its dose and note if any side effects (oxygen saturation, etc.)	
	Total (15)	

Kangaroo Mother Care

■ OBJECTIVE

The participants should be able to counsel the mother and family, initiate kangaroo mother care (KMC), and support the family to provide KMC, and monitor the infant during KMC.

■ SUPPLIES

- Cap
- Socks
- Disposable diaper
- Front-open sleeveless shirt
- KMC binder—long piece of cotton cloth/dupatta/KMC bag/KMC lycra bag **(Fig. 1)**.

■ STEPS

Counseling the mother and family:
- Greet the mother/family and make her comfortable.
- Explain about KMC including exclusive breastfeeding and encourage the family to ask questions **(Fig. 2)**.
- Instruct the mother to put on a front-opened top and on hand hygiene.
- Discuss how the family can support the mother in KMC.

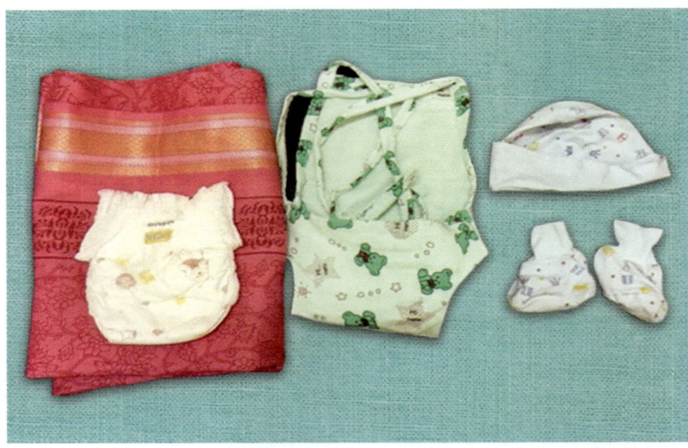

Fig. 1: Supplies required for KMC.

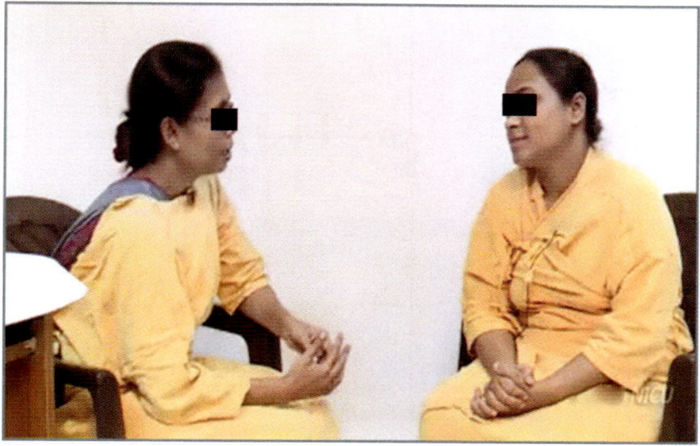

Fig. 2: Counsel and explain the mother about KMC.

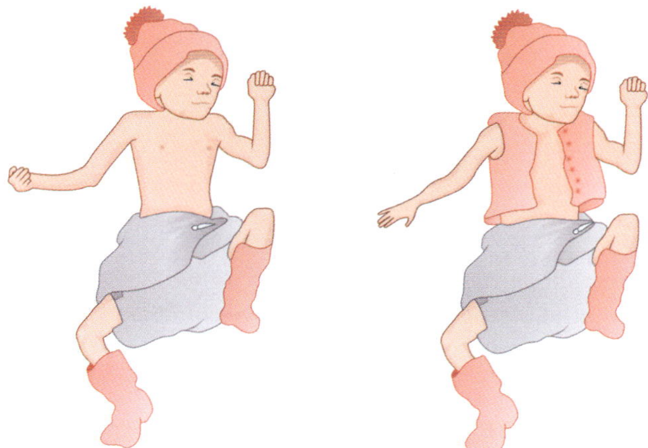

Fig. 3: Dressing the baby for KMC.

■ POSITIONING OF THE BABY AND THE MOTHER

- Dress the baby in diaper, cap, front open sleeveless shirt and socks **(Fig. 3)**.
- Place the baby between the mother's breasts in skin-to-skin contact on an upright position **(Fig. 4)**.
- Turn the head to one side with slight extension.
- Abduct the hips in a frog position and flex the arms **(Fig. 5)**.
- Support the baby's bottom with a sling/binder **(Fig. 6)**.
- Cover the baby with mother's gown.
- Show the mother how to move the baby in and out of the binder.
- Maintain a 30° recline by providing the mother with adjustable cots or reclining chairs **(Fig. 7)**.

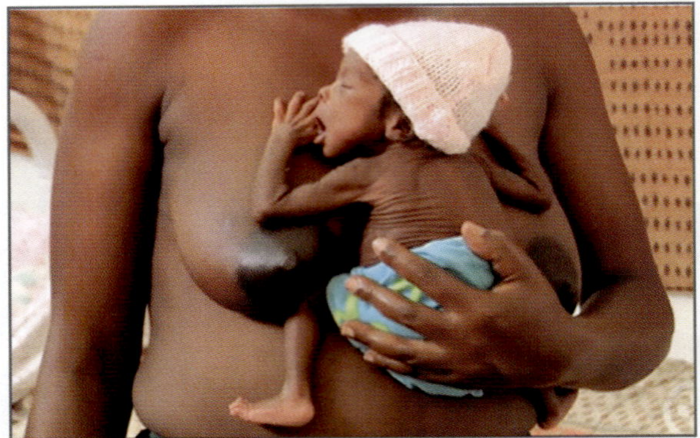

Fig. 4: Place the baby in between mothers' breasts, with head turned to one side

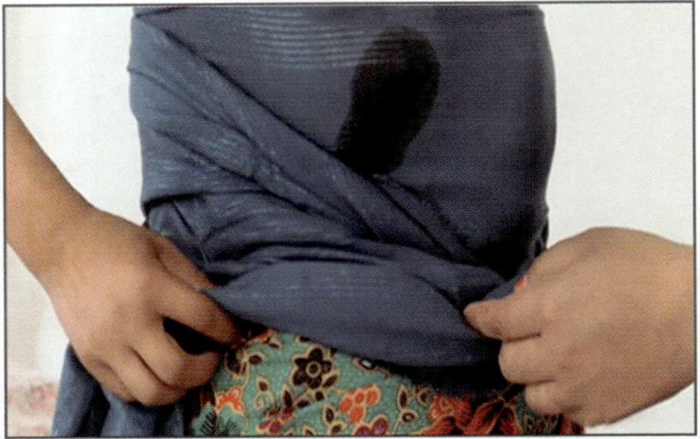

Fig. 5: Support the baby's bottom using a sling binder.

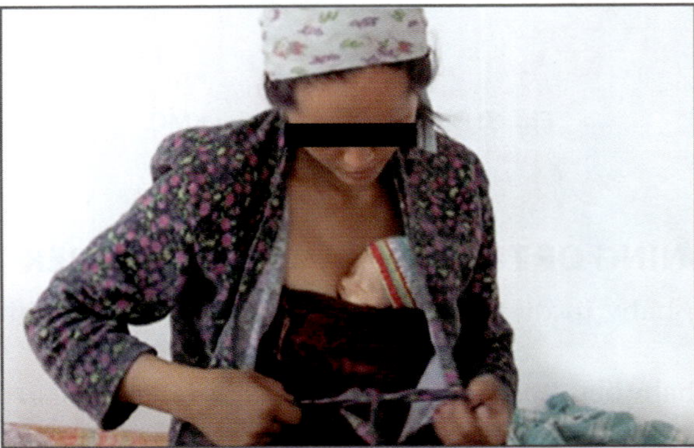

Fig. 6: Cover the baby with mother's gown.

■ MONITORING

- Monitor baby's activity, breathing, color, temperature **(Fig. 8)**.
- Use pulse oximeter, in very small or sick babies, if available **(Fig. 9)**.
- Monitor compliance to KMC and duration of KMC **(Fig. 10)**.

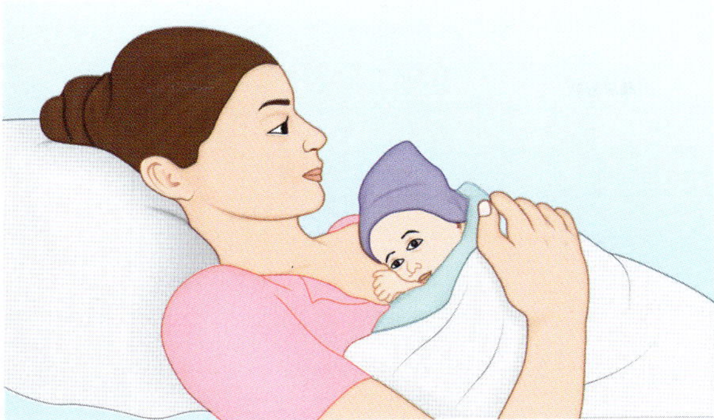

Fig. 7: Maintain a 30 degree recline.

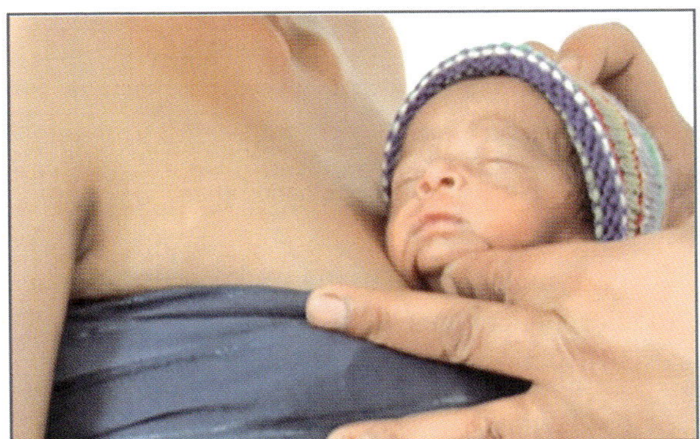

Fig. 8: Monitor baby's activity, colour, breathing and position of the neck

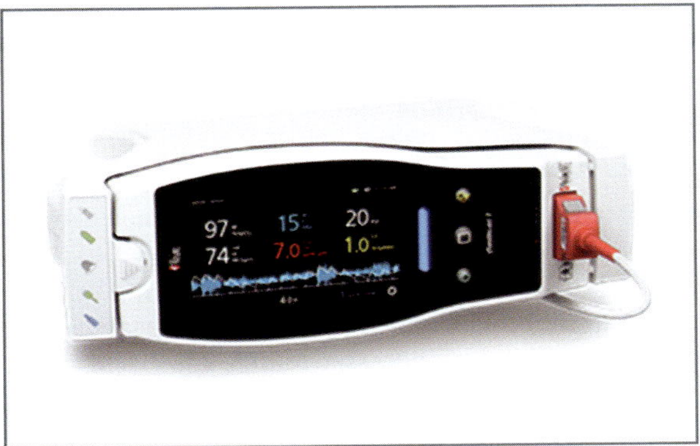

Fig. 9: Use pulse oximeter to monitor vitals.

■ DO'S ✅

- Start KMC as soon as possible after birth.
- Every KMC session should last at least 1 hour. The length of skin-to-skin contact should be as long as possible at least >8 hours/day.

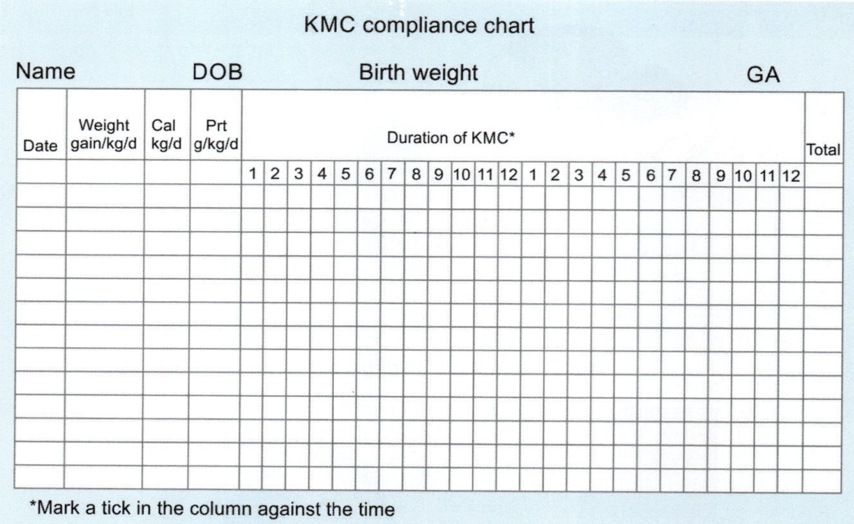

KMC compliance chart

Date	Weight gain/kg/d	Cal kg/d	Prt g/kg/d	Duration of KMC*																								Total
				1	2	3	4	5	6	7	8	9	10	11	12	1	2	3	4	5	6	7	8	9	10	11	12	

Name   DOB   Birth weight   GA

*Mark a tick in the column against the time

Fig. 10: KMC compliance chart.

- KMC provider carrying an infant in the KMC position can walk, stand, sit, or engage in different activities.
- Encourage exclusive mother's own milk feeds.

■ DON'T'S ❌

- Avoid frequent handling of the baby.
- Do not give bath to the baby till baby weighs 2,500 g.
- Do not give bottle feeds.
- Do not allow the baby to be in contact sick persons.

■ FURTHER READING

1. Global Health Media. Care of small babies (Keeping small baby warm). Available from: https://youtu.be/ecxLLUo71yo.
2. Hailegebriel T. (2018). Facilitators Guide for Training on Kangaroo Mother Care. Available from: https://www.healthynewbornnetwork.org/hnn-content/uploads/KMC-Guide.pdf [Last accessed March, 2024].
3. Ministry of Health and Family Welfare, Government of India. (2014). Kangaroo mother care and optimal feeding of the low birth weight infants: Operational guidelines. New Delhi: Child Health Division, Ministry of Health and Family Welfare; 2014.
4. Module 2: Kangaroo mother care. In: Facility-Based Care of Preterm Infant-Learner's guide [Internet]. First. New Delhi: AIIMS WHO–CC; 2018. Available from: https://www.newbornwhocc.org/Facility-Based-Care-of-Preterm-Infant.html.

TABLE 1: Objective structured clinical examination (OSCE) for kangaroo mother care (KMC).

S. No.	Steps	Points (1 each)
Counseling the mother:		
1.	Greets the mother	
2.	Sits at the same level and maintains eye contact	
3.	Asks the mother about the baby	
4.	Listens to her concerns	
5.	Praises the mother for her involvement in the care of the baby	
6.	Counsels the mother about KMC	
7.	Encourages the mother to ask questions	
8.	Instructs mother to put on a front-opened top	
Procedure:		
1.	Dresses the baby in diaper, cap, front open sleeveless shirt and socks	
2.	Places the baby between the mother's breasts in skin-to-skin contact on an upright position	
3.	Turns the head to one side with slight extension	
4.	Abducts the hips in a frog position and flex the arms	
5.	Supports the baby's bottom with a sling/binder	
6.	Covers the baby with mother's gown	
Monitoring:		
1.	Checks the position of the neck	
2.	Checks the temperature by touch method	
3.	Counts the respiratory rate by the chest movement	
4.	Checks the color of the baby/indicates the need for pulse oximeter if available	
5.	Advises mother how to monitor activity, breathing, color, temperature	
	Total (19)	

Retinopathy of Prematurity Screening

■ OBJECTIVE

The participants should be able to assist trained ophthalmologist in retinopathy of prematurity (ROP) screening of preterm infants efficiently and safely in a predesignated area of neonatal intensive care unit (NICU) or a follow-up clinic.

■ SUPPLIES AND EQUIPMENT

- Indirect ophthalmoscope (with small pupil adjustment)
- 20 D and 28 D condensing lenses for indirect ophthalmoscope
- Neonatal lid speculum also known as Alfonso eye speculum.
- Scleral indenter or depressor
- Dilating eye drops (tropicamide 0.5% + phenylephrine 2.5%)
- Artificial tears containing carboxymethyl cellulose
- Local anesthetic drops (proparacaine 0.5%)
- Consumables like sterile cotton swabs/wipes, and sterile gloves
- Hand wash/hand rub before the procedure
- Sterile tissues or towels for drying of hands.
- Clean baby sheets for swaddling and facilitated tuck (nonpharmacological pain control) as shown in **Figure 1**.
- Mother's expressed breast milk (EBM) soaked swab or 24% sucrose for pain control during the procedure.
- Pulse oximeter for monitoring.
- Functional resuscitation equipment (self-inflating bag, injection adrenaline, and normal saline)

■ PROCEDURE (PREPARATION AND ADMINISTRATION OF EYE DROPS) (BOX 1)

- Check patient list for the day.
- Counsel parents for the need of ROP screening procedure
- Preparation of eye drops **(Fig. 1)**
- Perform hand hygiene and put sterile gloves.
- Pull the lower palpebra to expose conjunctiva and administer one drop of diluted eye drops in the lower conjunctival sac and repeat this for the other eye.

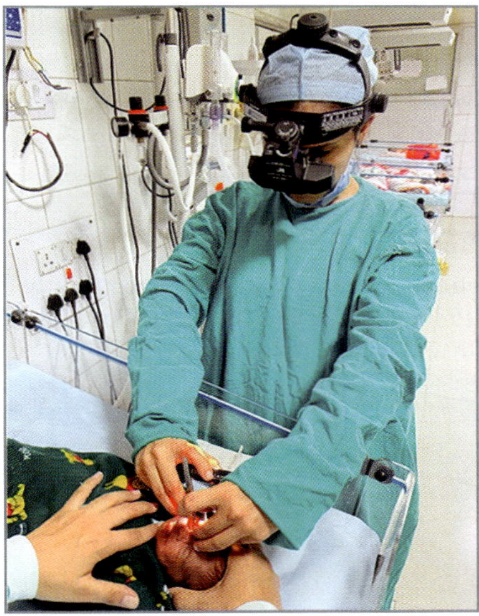

Fig. 1: Trained ophthalmologist performing retinopathy of prematurity (ROP) screening with proper nesting and facilitated tuck for pain control.

BOX 1: Preparation of eye drops for retinopathy of prematurity (ROP) screening.

Eye drops available in pharmacy:
- Tropicamide (0.8%)—phenylephrine (5%) combination: 5 mL vial (most commonly used used)
- Tropicamide (1%): 5 mL vial
- Phenylephrine (10%): 5 mL vial (not used nowadays)
- Tropicamide (0.8%)—phenylephrine (2.5%) combination (new): 5 mL vial

Recommended concentration to be used:
- Tropicamide: 0.5%
- Phenylephrine: 2.5% single dosage

Dilution:
- Tropicamide—phenylephrine combination: 1:1 dilution with carboxymethyl cellulose eye drops or distilled water
- Tropiamide: 1:1 dilution with carboxymethyl cellulose eye drops or distilled water

Dosage:
- Instill diluted combination drops or commercially available diluted drops three times every 10–15 minutes
- For nondiluting pupils suspect severe ROP

- Wipe the excess drug from medial to lateral side of the eye.
- Repeat the above two steps every 10 minutes for a total of three to four times.
- The pupil usually dilates within 30 minutes and remains dilated for 30–45 minutes.

- During the screening procedure, keep the baby well swaddled.
- For reducing pain, use nonpharmacological method like facilitated tuck or 24% sucrose/expressed breast milk (EBM)-soaked swab.
- Monitor the baby for 30–60 minutes post procedure for apnea and feed intolerance.

■ FURTHER READING

1. Singh A. Guidelines for Universal Eye screening in newborns including Retinopathy of Prematurity. New Delhi: Rashtriya Bal Swasthya Karyakram Ministry of Health and Family Welfare; 2017.

S. no.	Steps	Points (1 each)
TABLE 1: Objective structured clinical examination (OSCE) for retinopathy of prematurity (ROP) screening.		
1.	Counsels the parents for the need of ROP screening procedure	1
2.	Prepares the eye drops as per recommended dilution for the procedure	1
3.	Performs hand hygiene and put sterile gloves	1
4.	Pulls the lower palpebra to expose conjunctiva and administers one drop of diluted eye drops in the lower conjunctival sac and repeat this for the other eye	1
5.	Wipes the excess drug from the medial to lateral side of the eye	1
6.	Repeats the above two steps every 10 minutes for a total of three to four times	1
7.	During the screening procedure, keeps the baby well-swaddled.	1
8.	For reducing pain, uses nonpharmacological methods like facilitated tuck or 24% sucrose/expressed breast milk (EBM)-soaked swab	1
9.	Monitors the baby for 30–60 minutes post procedure for apnea and feed intolerance	1
	Total (9)	

Index

Page numbers followed by *b* refer to box, *f* refer to figure, and *t* refer to table.